Regenerative Injections in Sports Medicine

Suad Trebinjac • Manoj Kumar Nair

Regenerative Injections in Sports Medicine

An Evidenced Based Approach

Springer

Suad Trebinjac
CZECH Rehabilitation Hospital
Al Ain; FIFA Medical Center of Excellence
Dubai
United Arab Emirates

Manoj Kumar Nair
Dubai Health Authority
Dubai
United Arab Emirates

ISBN 978-981-15-6785-8 ISBN 978-981-15-6783-4 (eBook)
https://doi.org/10.1007/978-981-15-6783-4

This Springer imprint is published by the registered company Springer Nature Singapore Pte Ltd.
The registered company address is: 152 Beach Road, #21-01/04 Gateway East, Singapore 189721, Singapore

Foreword

As a professor neurosurgeon and the chairman of the Development Committee of the American Academy and Board of Regenerative Medicine, the Middle East and North Africa Chapter, I am honored and privileged to write a foreword for this important book in the field of regenerative medicine.

I consider Prof. Dr. Suad Trebinjac as one of the most active members in the MENA Chapter of the AABRM. He worked hard to finish all the requirements of the Diploma of the AABRM and deserved well to obtain it. He is a colleague and a friend from whom I get a lot of inspiration. We work together on many regenerative projects. He has recently been appointed as the Medical Director in one of the outstanding rehabilitation hospitals where he is working actively to establish an evidence-based regenerative therapy center. Dr. Manoj Kumar is another member of the MENA Chapter of the AABRM. We were part of the first group of doctors to prepare for the AABRM diploma. Since then, we have been close colleagues sharing the values of evidence-based regenerative practice. He is a known physician in his field, and his scientific approach is well appreciated by his patients and peers.

I am pleased that these important figures of regenerative medicine in the Middle East have written the book that will serve as a reference for biological therapy in the field of sports medicine. They have managed to cover all the important applications of regenerative medicine including prolotherapy. The latter is a subject that is often forgotten or missed in the arsenal of available therapies in regenerative medicine. It offers excellent results in a proper indication at a very moderate price. As we all know, the price of the treatment is an essential factor to decide on the availability and affordability of any treatment in every part of the world.

I feel that this book has contributed a great deal in filling the gap of evidence-based practice in the regenerative world. It is an important contribution made by these enthusiastic authors that will be an asset to doctors of the field not only in the Middle East but also all over the world.

As an expert in the field of regenerative medicine with particular interest in spinal pathologies, I have the pleasure of presenting this masterpiece to the medical and scientific community.

This book presents in a very well-illustrated method the wide indications of regenerative therapy in sports medicine. The book starts by defining regenerative medicine and the different types of regenerative treatment available. This paves the way for the reader to understand and digest the valuable content of the book. This is followed by another important chapter that discusses the mechanisms of injuries in sports. A presentation of the different regenerative therapies is then detailed in the following chapters. The rehabilitation part of this book stresses the importance of rehabilitation subsequent to regenerative treatment. So as a matter of fact, these two types of treatment go together and are complementary to each other. This solid clinical and scientific work is topped by the section on the future tendencies in biological therapies in sports medicine. In essence, this important work could be a guide for newly joining members to the community of biological therapy as well as for seasoned specialists to achieve perfection in their skills.

Both authors are highly experienced physical medicine and rehabilitation specialists with long and deep wealth of experience in the field of regenerative medicine. This makes them well capable of sharing this very interesting experience and knowledge with the sports medicine and the regenerative community.

In conclusion, I had a great joy in writing the foreword to this book as I believe that it is a valuable addition to the regenerative medicine library. It will be the companion and guide for orthopedics, sports medicine, rheumatologists, rehabilitation specialists, physiotherapists, and all regenerative practitioners in general in their daily practice. As the chairman of the Development Committee of the AABRM, I endorse strongly this masterpiece to my fellow readers written by these brilliant physicians. I would like to thank them sincerely for their tremendous efforts in completing this manuscript.

Liverpool, UK
London, UK
Dubai, UAE

Mohammed Al-Jumaily

Contents

About the Authors

Suad Trebinjac, MD, PhD, graduated from the Faculty of Medicine, University of Sarajevo, Bosnia and Herzegovina (former Yugoslavia). He is currently an Associate Professor at Dubai Medical College for Girls and Consultant on Physical Medicine and Rehabilitation to Al Garhoud Private Hospital/FIFA Medical Center of Excellence, Dubai, and CZECH Rehabilitation Hospital, Al Ain. Dr. Suad has more than 30 years of experience in the field of physiatry and 12 years of experience in prolotherapy and regenerative medicine.

Manoj Kumar Nair, MD, DNB, is certified by the National Board of Examinations India. Dr. Nair holds a Diploma in Sports Medicine from the International Olympic Committee and is currently working as a Specialist in Physical Medicine and Rehabilitation at the Dubai Health Authority. He has more than 15 years of experience as a specialist in Physical Medicine & Rehabilitation (Physiatry) and 5 years of experience in prolotherapy and regenerative medicine.

1 Introduction

After the definition of regenerative medicine, it is explained why it has become a very attractive medical discipline resulting in a huge number of published articles. The chapter is focused on three modalities that might have regenerative potential, they are dextrose prolotherapy, platelet-rich plasma (PRP), and mesenchymal stem cells. Different types of application of regenerative substances are mentioned, including injection to the ligaments, tendons, muscles, and joints, augmentation during the surgery, and through medical engineering.

Ethical dilemmas related to stem cells and alternative approaches to overcome such problems are suggested, by explaining potential and the advantages of induced pluripotent stem cells.

The importance of the application of regenerative substances in sports medicine is discussed, highlighting the benefit of this treatment compared to the classical therapeutic approach.

The literal meaning of the word regenerate is to create again. Regenerative medicine, by offering to create tissue and to cure, rather than to treat symptoms becomes a very attractive therapeutic scope for clinicians, researchers, and patients. It brings hope to millions of people suffering from chronic disorders. The number of research articles related to prolotherapy, platelet-rich plasma, and stem cells grew exponentially in the last 20 years. Preclinical and clinical studies enriched our knowledge and expertise, but also brought up certain controversies and sometimes disappointments.

Regenerative therapy already passed from animal studies to human applications and it made a footprint in different medical fields. One of them is sports medicine.

1.1 Definition of Regenerative Medicine

Despite growing interest, there is no consensus about the definition of regenerative medicine. Several proposals were suggested, including the one that regenerative medicine is a "process of replacing, engineering or regenerating human cells,

S. Trebinjac, M. K. Nair, *Regenerative Injections in Sports Medicine*,
https://doi.org/10.1007/978-981-15-6783-4_1

tissues or organs to restore or establish normal function" [1]. By stimulating the body's own mechanism, it offers the hope that impaired tissues will be eventually repaired and fully functional again. In a broad sense, it includes the possibility of growing tissues and organs in laboratory conditions with the potential of replacement of permanently impaired body structures. It would eventually solve the problem of transplanted organ rejection and shortage of organ donations [2].

1.2 Different Types of Regenerative Treatments

It is difficult to differentiate therapeutic procedures that have regenerative potential from purely symptomatic. The reason is a shortage of preclinical studies that can be reliably transferred to the paradigm of human clinical practice. It is known that results in vitro, as well as animal models, are not necessarily applicable to humans. Biological properties and mechanisms of action of certain procedures are not yet completely elucidated. Without well-designed randomized controlled trials, it will be difficult to differentiate between natural healing potential and healing stimulated by proliferative substances.

The ingredients with regenerative potential can be applied in different ways: by simple injections, as a part of surgical treatments, or by cells seeding of the scaffold. The last type of application belongs to the new scientific field called medical engineering [3]. There is no clear evidence which type of application is the most effective.

There are some ethical issues particularly related to embryonic stem cells and their use in many countries is strictly prohibited by law [4]. This is mainly because of the need to destroy an embryo and the concerns about the possibility of uncontrolled proliferation and the development of tumors. Teratoma and teratocarcinoma are well documented after transplantation of human embryonic stem cells to mice [5]. The law related to embryonic stem cells is applied to both research and clinical practice. Such issues are not relevant to the cells extracted from adults.

Japanese scientists were able to reprogram adult stem cells into embryonic-like cells. They are called induced pluripotent stem cells (iPSCs) [6]. These cells are the subject of intensive research due to their broader regenerative potential and high safety profile.

While recognizing that different substances might have proliferative potential and can get prefix regenerative, we decided to present the three most common therapeutic procedures considered as a part of regenerative medicine- they are dextrose prolotherapy, platelet-rich plasma (PRP), and mesenchymal stem cells. Our research is limited to injection-based therapy only.

1.3 Importance of Regenerative Medicine in Sport

Over the last century, interest in the field of sports medicine has been growing all over the world. This is partially due to increased awareness of healthy living, but also due to driving force pertinent to young people to compete and to prove themselves.

There is an increase in the number of young people choosing sports as their profession. For professional athletes, good health and fitness are of paramount importance. Unfortunately, injuries are an inescapable part of the sport.

Their incidence, prevalence, and type vary among both genders and different age groups [7]. Soft tissue injuries including muscles, tendons, and ligaments are very common. Excessive mechanical load causes structural changes inside the tissues provoking pain and limited function. It is documented that tendon stretches of 4%–8% elicit microscopic damages and beyond 12% can cause a total rupture [8]. Repetitive stress and overuse can cause microscopic changes in tendons making them more weak and susceptible to failure [9]. Exercise increase vascularity of tendons and muscles, synthesis of collagen,but also activation of matrix metalloproteinases, protein degrading enzymes. Activation of these enzymes explaines pathogenesis of tendon injuries [10]. Other factors like age, poor vascular supply, and genetic factors contribute to the development of tendinopathies even in less physically active people [11].

An injured player wants to return back to the playground as soon as possible. Prolonged rest deteriorates physical condition, diminishes performance skills, and causes mental stress, anxiety, and depression. It is found that even a short rest of fewer than 10 days produces a decrease in lean mass, reducing one repetition maximum muscle power, diminishing cross-sectional area of quadriceps, and reducing insulin sensitivity accompained by reduction of muscle oxidative capacity [12]. The metabolism of tendons and ligaments is much slower than muscles, hence the healing process is more delayed [13].

The major goal of physicians dealing with athletes is to restore the pre-injury level of function in the shortest possible period of time without compromising the natural healing process [14]. It is understandable considering that unhealed injuries affect optimal performance and ruin their professional career.

The treatment of sports injuries was traditionally symptomatic. The golden rule for acute injuries was summarized in the acronym RICE (rest, ice, compression, and elevation). Short-term immobilization and the use of anti-inflammatory medications can be added [15]. This approach, while reducing the symptoms, does not stimulate the regenerative process needed for functional recovery. Animal studies show that reducing neutrophils and leukocytes as inflammatory mediators do not increase the function and strength of tendons. Consequently, nonsteroidal anti-inflammatory drugs (NSAID) will not promote better healing [16]. On the contrary, studies in animals show that COX 2 inhibitors impair the physiological healing process in ligaments of rats by inhibiting fibroblast growth [17].

Prolonged rest and early mobilization, both might have a negative impact on natural recovery. Atrophy of muscles from rest and immobilization and scar tissue due to early mobilization [18] are physiological consequences of wrongly applied RICE concept. Unfortunately, clinical practice is full of such examples. Many players are in a hurry to return back to training, while others are interested in longer rest than needed.

The psychological effect of sports injuries is significant, and it is manifested with low mood, frustration, and depression. Some people feel tired, confused, and bored [19]. It affects results in both competitive and recreational sports. The economic burden related to the management of sports injuries is difficult to estimate because of uncertain incidence and prevalence [7].

The concept of regenerative medicine is useful in musculoskeletal conditions because its application accelerates the healing process. It is particularly important considering the chronicity and slow healing as a typical feature of tendon and ligament injuries common among athletes. In professional sport, time means money, and return to play is the matter of profit, not only of personal pleasure.

The application of regenerative ingredients is sometimes the only alternative to surgical treatment, which is aggressive, risky, and more expensive. The new concept of orthobiologics and regenerative medicine is aimed at reducing open surgeries, by injecting regenerative substances whenever it is possible [20].

Key Points

- Regenerative medicine is fast-growing medical discipline finding its place.

  In sports medicine.

- Three injection-based therapeutic modalities with possible regenerative potential are dextrose prolotherapy, platelet-rich plasma, and mesenchymal stem cells.
- Embryonic stem cells possess big regenerative potential but their use is unethical and potentially dangerous. Reprogramming adult stem cells into embryo-like cells might be a good solution in the future.
- Traditional treatment of sports injuries is symptom-oriented and does not stimulate complete restitution of injured tissues.
- Regenerative injections could speed up the healing process and provide better therapeutic outcomes. It can be a good alternative to surgical treatment.

References

1. Mason C, Dunnill P. A brief definition of regenerative medicine. Regen Med. 2008 Jan 1;3(1):1–5.
2. Regenerative medicine glossary. Regen Med. 2009 July;4(4 Suppl):S1–88.
3. Ouyang HW, Goh JCH, XM M, SH T, EH L. The efficacy of bone marrow stromal cell-seeded knitted PLGA fiber scaffold for Achilles tendon repair. Ann N Y Acad Sci. 2002 Jun;961(1):126–9.
4. Robertson JA. Science and society: human embryonic stem cell research: ethical and legal issues. Nat Rev Genet. 2001 Jan 1;2(1):74.
5. Hentze H, Soong PL, Wang ST, Phillips BW, Putti TC, Dunn NR. Teratoma formation by human embryonic stem cells: evaluation of essential parameters for future safety studies. Stem Cell Res. 2009;2(3):198–210.
6. Takahashi K, Yamanaka S. Induction of pluripotent stem cells from mouse embryonic and adult fibroblast cultures by defined factors. Cell. 2006;126(4):663–76.
7. Öztürk S. What is the economic burden of sports injuries? Joint Diseases and Related Surg. 2013 Aug 20;24(2):108–11.
8. Wang JH. Mechanobiology of a tendon. J Biomech. 2006;39(9):1563–82.

9. Kirkendall DT, Garrett WE. Function and biomechanics of tendons. Scand J Med Sci Sports. 1997 Apr;7(2):62–6.
10. Kjær M, Magnusson P, Krogsgaard M, Møller JB, Olesen J, Heinemeier K, et al. Extracellular matrix adaptation of tendon and skeletal muscle to exercise. J Anat. 2006 Apr;208(4):445–50.
11. Young JS, Kumta SM, Maffulli N. Achilles tendon rupture and Tendinopathy: management of complications. Foot Ankle Clin. 2005;10(2):371–82.
12. Dirks ML, Wall BT, van de Valk B, Holloway TM, Holloway GP, Chabowski A, et al. One week of bed rest leads to substantial muscle atrophy and induces whole-body insulin resistance in the absence of skeletal muscle lipid accumulation. Diabetes. 2016 Oct;65(10):2862–75.
13. Zernicke RF, Garhammer J, Jobe FW. Human patellar-tendon rupture. J Bone Joint Surg. 1977 Mar;59(2):179–83.
14. Warden SJ. Cyclo-Oxygenase-2 inhibitors: beneficial or detrimental for athletes with acute musculoskeletal injuries? Sports Med. 2005;35(4):271–83.
15. Järvinen TAH, Järvinen TLN, Kääriäinen M, Äärimaa V, Vaittinen S, Kalimo H, Järvinen M. Muscle injuries: optimizing recovery. Best Pract Res Clin Rheumatol. 2007;21(2):317–31.
16. Marsolais D, Côté CH, Frenette J. Nonsteroidal anti-inflammatory drug reduces neutrophil and macrophage accumulation but does not improve tendon regeneration. Lab Investig. 2003 Jul;83(7):991–9.
17. Elder CL, Dahners LE, Weinhold PS. A Cyclooxygenase-2 inhibitor impairs ligament healing in the rat. Am J Sports Med. 2001 Nov 1;29(6):801–5.
18. Järvinen MJ, Lehto MU. The effects of early mobilization and immobilization on the healing process following muscle injuries. Sports Med. 1993 Feb;15(2):78–89.
19. Pearson L, Jones G. Emotional effects of sports injuries: implications for physiotherapists. Physiotherapy. 1992;78(10):762–70.
20. Sampson S, Botto-van Bemden A, Aufiero D. Autologous bone marrow concentrate: review and application of a novel intra-articular orthobiologic for cartilage disease. Phys Sportsmed. 2013 Sep;41(3):7–18.

Injury Mechanisms in Sports

2

This chapter highlights the increasing prevalence of sports injuries and negative long-term effects on active players. It emphasized the importance of recognizing intrinsic and extrinsic factors responsible for the onset of injuries and their severity. While planning the training, individual variations and gender differences should be considered along with physiological changes due to aging process. Prevention of sports injury starts with an analysis of all elements that might predict their development. A four-step prevention plan is suggested to minimize the negative consequences. Mechanisms of injuries specific to different sports are highlighted.

The annual rate of sports-related injuries among high school athletes was estimated to be around two million in 2005–2006 with 500,000 doctor visits and 30,000 hospital admissions [1]. Some of them have serious consequences for athletes. Aside from the loss of time and treatment expenses they can lead to long-term tissue impairment. One such example is secondary knee osteoarthritis developing in almost all people 15–20 years after the injury [2].

Sports injuries are the result of the interplay of multiple factors that might be biochemical and mechanical. Why some athletes are at risk of injury depends on different intrinsic and extrinsic factors as well as on inciting events that are critical for tissue impairment [3]. Among the important intrinsic factors are age, sex, and body composition, while extrinsic factors might be related to the quality of the playground (wet floor), climate, inadequate footwear, or clothes, poor coaching, etc. The example of inciting events are landing on the knee in valgus position (risk for the tear of an anterior cruciate ligament—ACL) or direct contact with the opposite player (Fig. 2.1).

Aging is a biological process that has a great impact on the musculoskeletal system. The density of bone is reduced, cartilage volume is decreased, the elasticity of muscles, ligaments, and tendons decline. Female body composition is different from male and less resistant to external stress. Changes in body structure and biomechanics are directly responsible for the severity of injury because any abnormalities in the mentioned features make the body more vulnerable. In such conditions,

S. Trebinjac, M. K. Nair, *Regenerative Injections in Sports Medicine*,
https://doi.org/10.1007/978-981-15-6783-4_2

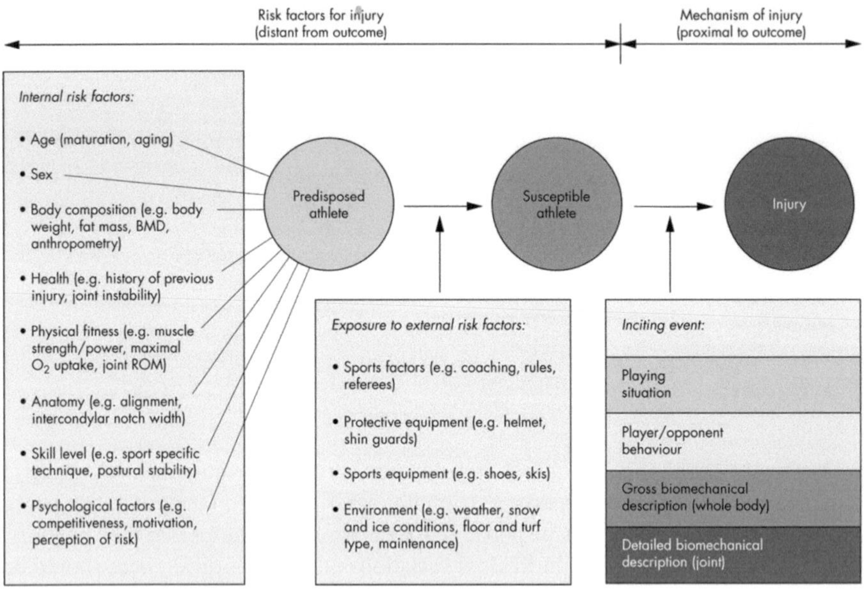

Fig. 2.1 Factors involved in the development of sports injuries from [4] with permission

the lower mechanical load and transfer of energy might be more detrimental than higher load imposed to physiologically sound body structures.

Extrinsic factors might increase or decrease the risk of injury. For example, poorly maintained football pitch can cause frequent inversion of the ankle joint or pivotal movements of the knee with the fixed foot. Both positions will increase the load and elicit damage to ligaments and tendons. On the other hand, appropriate clothes or equipment can protect the body from injury. The good examples are shin guards in football players, helmets in skiing, or rugby or mouth guards in boxing. However, external protection of the body might cause overconfidence in athletes, prompting them to expose their bodies to the additional load. It will result in injury, causing concern about the real benefit of protective equipment [5].

While intrinsic factors are the most important for the load tolerance, triggering events determine the load intensity and onset of the injury. In sports like football, basketball, and handball contact with opponents, landing, cutting, pivoting are the most common events which transfer mechanical energy to tissue. Disbalance between load intensity and load tolerance are crucial factors in the development of injury.

Additional modifiable factors, like attitude, motivation, and training skills also increase or decrease the risk.

Obviously, the selection of sport is one of the most important factors determining the frequency and severity of injuries. While football and handball players get one injury in 10 matches, volleyball players will get one in 100 [6].

Prevention of injuries is the main objective of health professionals participating in sports care. It is based on four parts complementary to each other [3] (Fig. 2.2).

Fig. 2.2 Four-step sequence of injury prevention [3]

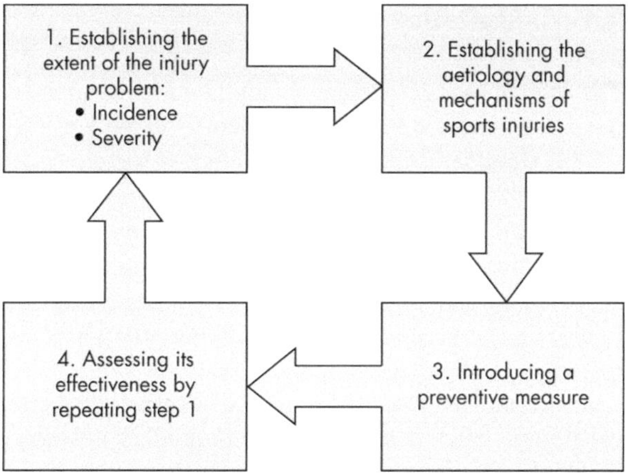

To formulate a robust sports injury prevention program, a better understanding of the elements involved in injury development is essential. The plan has to be specific for different types of injuries and in a broad sense to different sports. Consideration of intrinsic factors is an important element in formulating the program, as aging produces changes in the properties of tissues. Lack of muscle power, strength, endurance, balance, and coordination can be rectified through appropriate training. Foot deformities could be corrected by appropriate orthotic appliances. Other protective equipment should be used whenever needed.

Triggering factors of injury present combination of biomechanical properties (rotation of the leg, extreme abduction, foot inversion or eversion, etc.), player action (running, landing to one leg, falling down, etc.), the action of the opponent player (stepping on the opponent's foot, direct contact including hit by an elbow to the ribs, head to head contact, etc.).To avoid injuries caused by the action of other players strict rules with clear restrictions must be implemented and violation adequately sanctioned.

A proper selection of young people for certain sports categories is one of the key factors in the prevention of injuries. A genetic factor is another element to be considered as it has an impact on body constitution and natural talent. In addition to it, factors like positive attitude, motivation, and psychological status also influence the severity of the injury.

Analysis of modifiable factors and steps taken to correct them, backed up by scientific evidence is needed to make sure the implemented measures are having the desired results.

Different sports activities make certain parts of the body more vulnerable. Generally, upper limbs are more affected in boxing, tennis, volleyball, handball, baseball, while lower limbs are more afftected in football, running and jumping.

In the following section, a brief descripton of common mechanisms of injuries related to different joints are presented.

2.1 Shoulder

The shoulder is a very complex joint consisting of three bones, four joints, and eight muscles connected between ligaments and tendons—Fig. 2.3.

The shoulder joint is prone to injuries because it is the most mobile joint in the human body [7]. Its instability is counteracted by rotator cuff muscles, ligaments, tendons, and glenoid labrum [8]. Overhead movements and direct contact with other players are the most common causing factors of injuries among athletes [9]. In sports like baseball, volleyball, swimming, javelin throw, and handball, shoulder injuries are common, when stabilizing structures are overloaded by accelerated movements (Fig. 2.4).

It is estimated that around 57% of baseball pitchers suffer some types of a shoulder injury, which is much more than in other position players. Common pathology includes rotator cuff tear, superior labral anterior-posterior (SLAP), internal impingement, and microtrauma [10]. Repetitive injuries are followed by joint instability and limited function [11].

In contact sports, the pathology is a bit different. The study conducted on elite college football players revealed the most frequent shoulder injuries were acromioclavicular separation (41%), followed by anterior instability (20%), rotator cuff injury (12%), clavicle fracture (4%), and posterior instability (4%). The majority of injuries are due to contact with other players or playing surface [12]. Reduced shoulder movements, muscle atrophy, and weakness, as well as scapular dyskinesis, have been associated with more frequent shoulder injuries [13].

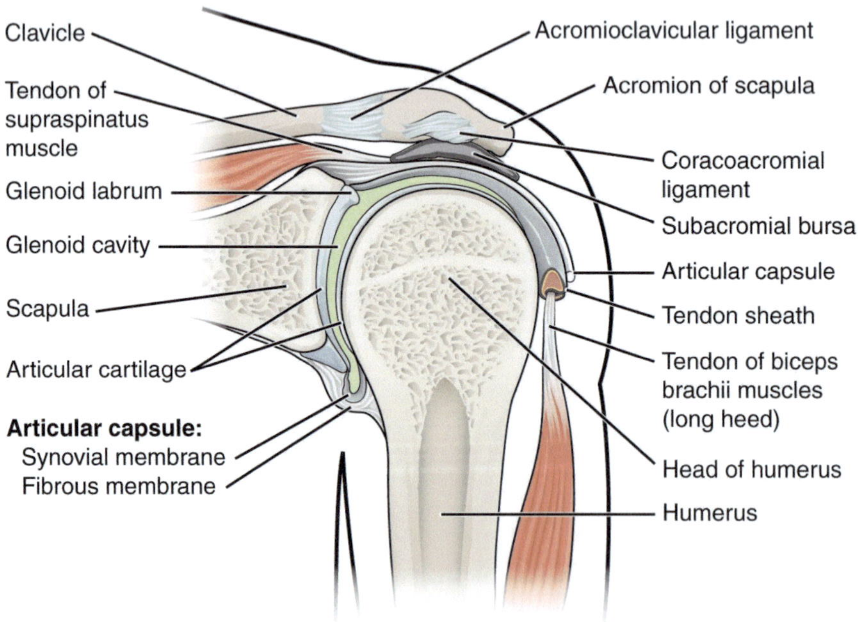

Fig. 2.3 Basic anatomy of the shoulder joint. From Wikimedia Commons OpenStax College

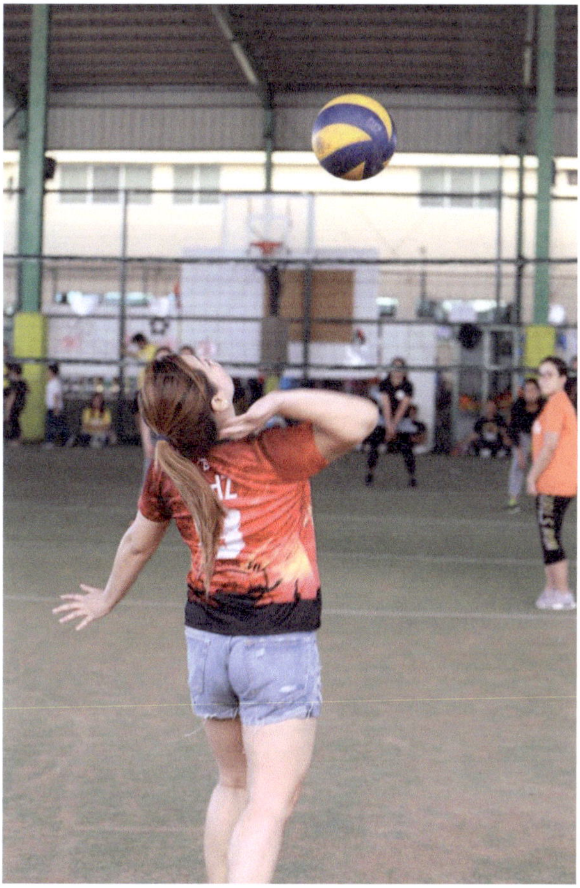

Fig. 2.4 Overstretch of shoulder joint. Image Courtesy Mr. Glendale Alkuino

2.2 Elbow

Elbow is a hinged joint consisting of three bones, humerus, radius, and ulna. It is connected with two major ligament medial and lateral collateral ligaments that provide main stability to the joint (Fig. 2.5).

The injuries are common in racquet sports, golf, weight lifting, and throwing. Muscles, tendons, and ligaments are usual sources of pain.

Lateral epicondylitis (tennis elbow) is the most frequent elbow injury and it is present in more than 50% of athletes practicing overhead arm movements [14]. Usually, it is developed by repetitive stress eliciting micro traumatic injuries to the extensors attached to the lateral epicondyle. Improper technique and inadequate equipment (too heavy a racquet) are the triggering factors (Fig. 2.6).

The second most common injury is medial epicondylitis (golfer's elbow). It accounts for 10–20% of all epicondylitis [15]. In both cases, tendons attaching to epicondyles are involved in the pathological process. The ulnar collateral ligament injury is only rarely encountered prolotherapy.

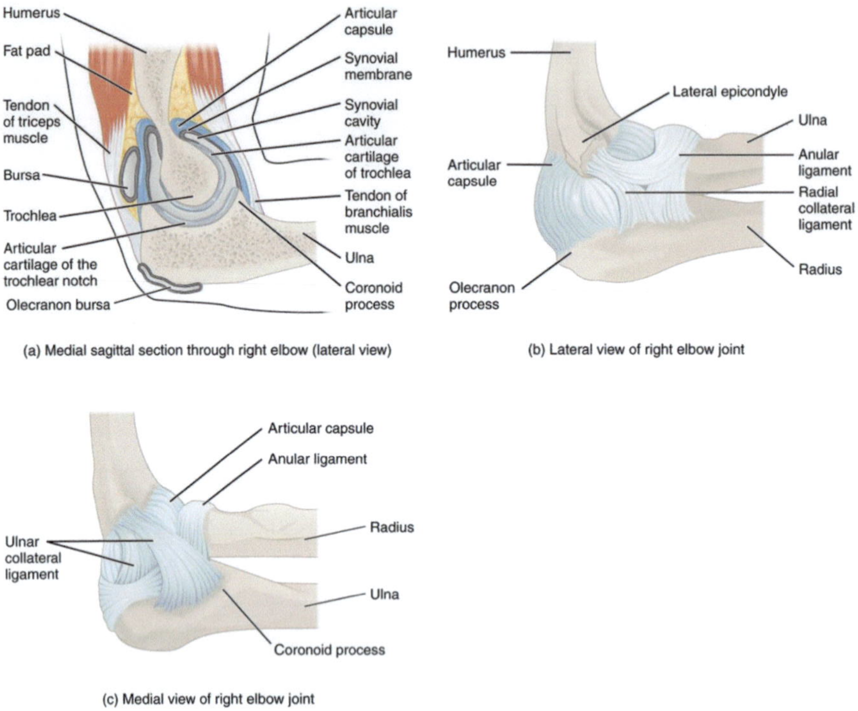

Fig. 2.5 Basic anatomy of elbow joint. From Wikimedia Commons OpenStax College

Fig. 2.6 Lateral epicondylitis (tennis elbow) can be caused by improper technique and heavy racquet. Image Courtesy Mr. Glendale Alkuino

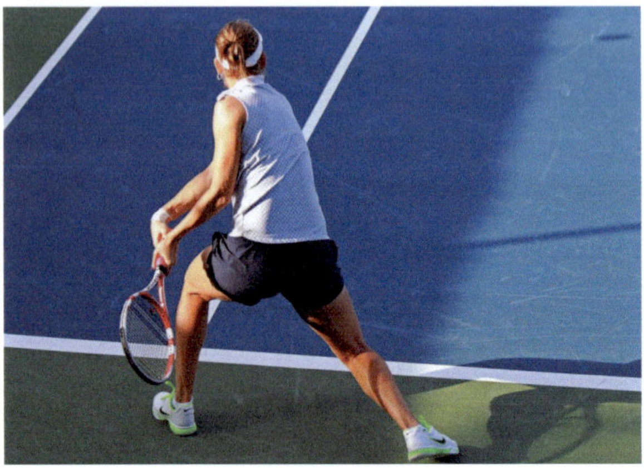

2.3 Wrist and Hand

It is estimated that up to 25% of the total number of sports injuries involve the wrist or hand [16]. A scaphoid fracture is a common and unpleasant injury [17]. The mechanism of injury is mainly related to pronated and hyperextended wrist radial deviation. Falling on an outstretched hand is the most common cause (Fig. 2.7). Scapholunate ligament is the most frequently injured carpal ligament causing instability in a joint [18]. The triangular fibrocartilaginous complex is a specific injury on the ulnar side and it is commonly caused by repetitive injuries in athletes [19]. Other ligaments and tendons are also frequently affected.

2.4 Hip and Groin

Hip and groin pain are common in athletes involved in cutting, pivoting, and kicking activities during sports performance. They are frequently observed in soccer and hockey players [20] (Fig. 2.8).

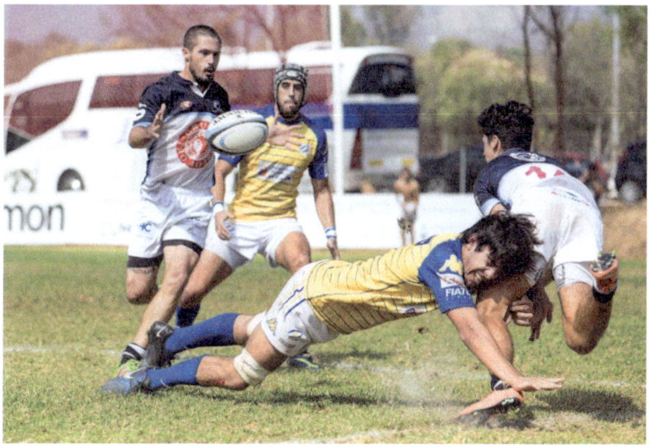

Fig. 2.7 Wrist extension and radial deviation—the most common mechanism of scaphoid fracture. Photo by Quino Al on Unsplash

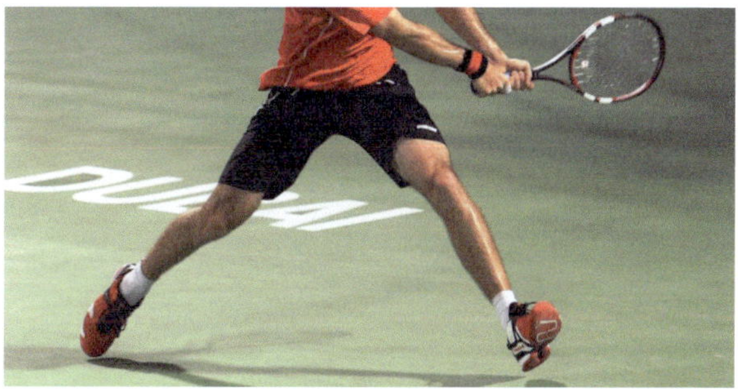

Fig. 2.8 A common mechanism of adductor and groin injuries overstretched leg. Image Courtesy Mr. Glendale Alkuino

Considering that different anatomical structures can cause pain in the groin and hip area, precise terminology and definition were necessary to avoid ambiguous diagnoses. The group of experts in the meeting in Doha, 2014 reach an agreement and divided hip/groin injuries into three categories:

- Adductor-related, iliopsoas-related, inguinal-related, and pubic-related groin pain
- Hip-related groin pain
- Other causes of groin pain in athletes [21].

Previous groin injuries, high level of play, reduced hip adductor strength, and lower levels of sports specific training are the main risk factors for injuries [22].

2.5 Knee

After the ankle, a knee is the most frequently injured joint in athletes and the most frequently operated [4]. Among US high school sportsmen, football has the highest knee injury rate [23], and some of them can end their professional career [24].

ACL tear is the most common injury in football, basketball, and volleyball, while meniscus injury is the most frequent in street runners [25]. The ACL injury occurs usually without contact with other players. A sudden change of direction followed by deceleration, hyperextension, and rotation of the leg is a common mechanism of injury (Fig. 2.9).

2.6 Ankle and Foot

Ankle and foot injuries are the most common injuries in athletes [26]. According to research on the US high school sports players, the rate of ankle and foot injuries accounted for 22.6% of all injuries. The highest risk was among athletes

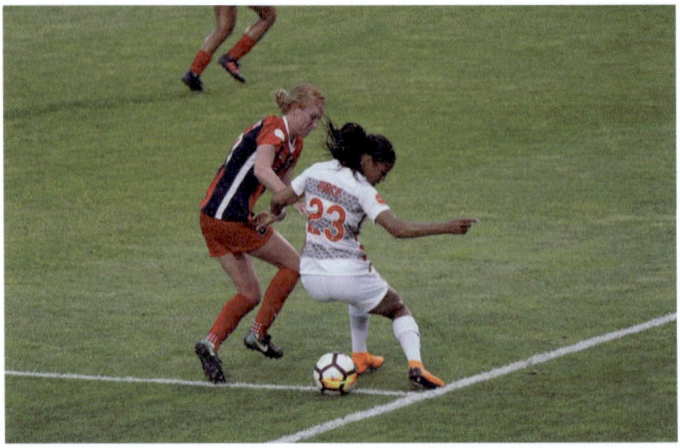

Fig. 2.9 The typical position of the knee during the ACL injury. Photo by Jeffrey F Lin on Unsplash

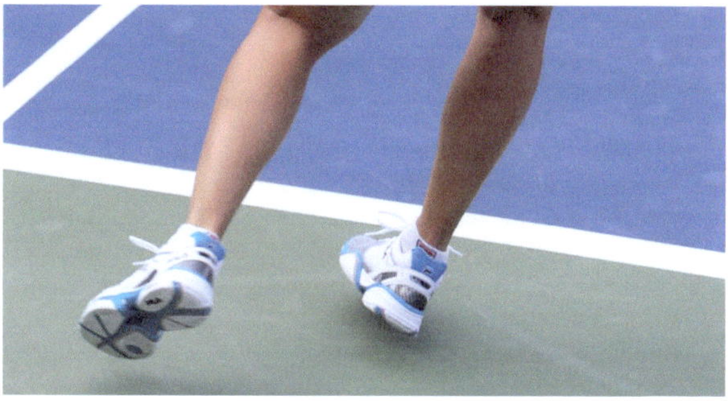

Fig. 2.10 Lateral ankle sprain—the most common type of ankle–foot injury. Image Courtesy Mr. Glendale Alkuino

participating in sports involving jumping and swift changes in direction as in basketball, football, and volleyball [26].

A sprain is the most common type of injury, and the anterior talofibular ligament is the most frequently affected structure [26, 27] (Fig. 2.10). It is estimated that around 70% of patients experience repetitive lateral ankle sprain injury causing chronic symptoms and joint instability [28].

Key Points

- The number of sports injuries increasing all over the world. Some of them seriously provoking long-term functional impairment and chronic pain.
- The interplay of different intrinsic and extrinsic factors contribute to the development of sports injuries.
- The prevention injury model consists of four parts complementary to each other. It is based on an analysis of all modifiable factors which might elicit tissue damage.
- Different sports cause different types and locations of injuries. Accordingly, an individual therapeutic plan has to be implemented.

References

1. Comstock RD, Yard E, Gilchrist J, Knox C. Sports-related injuries among high school athletes–United States, 2005-06 school year. MMWR Morb Mortal Wkly Rep. 2006 Sep 29;55(38):1037.
2. Myklebust G, Bahr R. Return to play guidelines after anterior cruciate ligament surgery. Br J Sports Med. 2005 Mar;39(3):127–31.
3. Bahr R, Krosshaug T. Understanding injury mechanisms: a key component of preventing injuries in sport. Br J Sports Med. 2005 Jun;39(6):324–9.
4. Joseph AM, Collins CL, Henke NM, Yard EE, Fields SK, Comstock RD. A multisport epidemiologic comparison of anterior cruciate ligament injuries in high school athletics. J Athl Train. 2013 Nov;48(6):810–7.
5. McIntosh AS. Risk compensation, motivation, injuries, and biomechanics in competitive sport. Br J Sports Med. 2005 Jan;39(1):2–3.
6. Bahr R, Kannus P, Van Mechelen W. Epidemiology and prevention of sports injuries. In: Textbook of Sports Medicine. Oxford, UK: Blackwell Science Ltd; 2008. p. 299–314.

7. Quillen DM, Wuchner M, Hatch RL. Acute shoulder injuries. Am Fam Physician. 2004 Nov 15;70(10):1947.
8. Jenkins DB. Hollinshead's functional anatomy of the limbs and Back. 9th ed. Saint Louis: Elsevier; 2008.
9. Krishnan SG. The shoulder and the overhead athlete. 1st ed. Philadelphia, PA; London: Lippincott Williams & Wilkins; 2004.
10. Ouellette H, Ouellette H, Labis J, Labis J, Bredella M, Bredella M, et al. Spectrum of shoulder injuries in the baseball pitcher. Skelet Radiol. 2008 Jun;37(6):491–8.
11. Pujalte GGA, Zaslow TL. A practical guide to shoulder injuries in the throwing athlete. J Fam Pract. 2013 Apr;62(4):175.
12. Kaplan LD, Flanigan DC, Norwig J, Jost P, Bradley J. Prevalence and variance of shoulder injuries in elite collegiate football players. Am J Sports Med. 2005 Aug 1;33(8):1142–6.
13. Clarsen B, Bahr R, Andersson SH, Munk R, Myklebust G. Reduced glenohumeral rotation, external rotation weakness and scapular dyskinesis are risk factors for shoulder injuries among elite male handball players: a prospective cohort study. Br J Sports Med. 2014 Sep;48(17):1327–33.
14. Field LD, Savoie FH. Common elbow injuries in sport. Sports Med. 1998 Sep;26(3):193–205.
15. Descatha AR, Shiri E, Viikari-Juntura H, Varonen M. Heliövaara Prévalence et déterminants des épicondylites latérale et médiales: une enquête en population générale Prevalence and determinants of lateral and medial epicondylitis: a population study Am J Epidemiol 164 2006 1065 1074. Archives des Maladies Professionnelles et de l'Environnement. 2007;68(5):586.
16. Lee SW. Musculoskeletal injuries and conditions. New York: Demos Medical Publishing; 2016.
17. Sendher R, Ladd AL. The scaphoid. Orthop Clin N Am. 2013;44(1):107–20.
18. Andersson JK. Treatment of scapholunate ligament injury: current concepts. EFORT Open Reviews. 2017 Sep;2(9):382–93.
19. Nagle DJ. Triangular fibrocartilage complex tears in the athlete. Clin Sports Med. 2001;20(1):155–66.
20. Topol GA, Reeves KD. Regenerative injection of elite athletes with career-altering chronic groin pain who fail conservative treatment: a consecutive case series. Am J Phys Med Rehabil. 2008 Nov;87(11):890–902.
21. Weir A, Brukner P, Delahunt E, Ekstrand J, Griffin D, Khan KM, et al. Doha agreement meeting on terminology and definitions in groin pain in athletes. Br J Sports Med. 2015 Jun;49(12):768–74.
22. Whittaker JL, Small C, Maffey L, Emery CA. Risk factors for groin injury in sport: an updated systematic review. Br J Sports Med. 2015 Jun;49(12):803–9.
23. Swenson DM, Collins CL, Best TM, Flanigan DC, Fields SK, Comstock RD. Epidemiology of knee injuries among U.S. high school athletes, 2005/2006–2010/2011. Med Sci Sports Exerc. 2013 Mar;45(3):462–9.
24. Engström B, Forssblad M, Johansson C, Tornkvist H. Does a major knee injury definitely sideline an elite soccer player? Am J Sports Med. 1990 Jan 1;18(1):101–5.
25. Nicolini AP, de Carvalho RT, Matsuda MM, Sayum JF, Cohen M. Common injuries in athletes' knee: experience of a specialized center. Acta Ortopedica Brasileira. 2014;22(3):127–31.
26. Nelson AJ, Collins CL, Yard EE, Fields SK, Comstock RD. Ankle injuries among United States high school sports athletes, 2005-2006. J Athl Train. 2007 Jul;42(3):381–7.
27. Ferran NA, Maffulli N. Epidemiology of sprains of the lateral ankle ligament complex. Foot Ankle Clin. 2006;11(3):659–62.
28. McKay GD, Goldie PA, Payne WR, Oakes BW. Ankle injuries in basketball: injury rate and risk factors. Br J Sports Med. 2001;35(2):103–8.

3 Current Practices in Sports Injury Rehabilitation

Well-structured rehabilitation programs are essential in return to sports of the injured athlete. This chapter touches upon the current concepts in sports injury management and 4 stages of sports rehabilitation. It also gives a brief about the theoretical approaches for adhering to a rehabilitation program.

Rehabilitation after sports injuries is essential for a timely and safe return to sports (RTS) activities. The goal of the rehabilitation program is to restore preinjury function, even though it is not practical to achieve in all athletes. Improper rehabilitation or premature entry into sporting activities can result in detrimental effects for the athletes, as this may predispose for reinjuries and turn an innocuous injury to a sinister one.

Any tissue damage results in pain and swelling and in addition produce effusion in joints. The basic doctrine of managing any sports injury is by the RICE principle. RICE is an acronym for rest, ice, compression, and elevation. Over the years, various modifications are suggested in this basic principle. It has changed to PRICE, by the addition of "protection" to the RICE principle. Lately, the concept has changed to POLICE, which stands for protection, optimal loading, ice, compression, and elevation [1].

There are no uniformly accepted protocols in sports injury rehabilitation and protocols and programs should be individualized to the specific patient needs.

General principles of any sports rehabilitation program should aim to achieve the following goals: [2].

- Reducing pain
- Reducing the edema
- Restoration of range of movement
- Regaining sports-specific muscle strength
- Normalizing motor control
- Improving the gait and close kinetic chain motion
- Improving proprioceptive deficits
- Controlled loading and return to impact activities

S. Trebinjac, M. K. Nair, *Regenerative Injections in Sports Medicine*,
https://doi.org/10.1007/978-981-15-6783-4_3

- Minimizing reinjury risk
- Sport-specific agility drills
- Maintaining cardiovascular fitness
- Address any intrinsic and extrinsic factors

Generally speaking, there are 4 stages involved in sports rehabilitation.

- Stage 1:
  It starts with the PRICE/ POLICE principle. When the athlete does not have pain, swelling, effusion, and having a full range of movement, he can progress to the stage 2.
- Stage 2:
  The main activities of this stage are open, closed kinetic exercises, proprioceptive exercises, and running. If an athlete does not have pain, swelling, effusion, and recovers full strength can progress to stage 3.
- Stage 3:
  This stage focuses on sports-specific drills and reconditioning. When the athlete gains sport-specific skills and has no pain, swelling, and effusion can progress to the final stage of rehabilitation.
- Stage 4:
  The main aims of this stage are the maintenance and prevention of reinjury. When the athlete maintains the conditioning he is certified as having full functional recovery and completes the rehabilitation program.

During any of these stages, if the athlete develops pain, swelling, or effusion, he drops back to the previous stage and repeats the program.

These stages are summarized in Fig. 3.1.

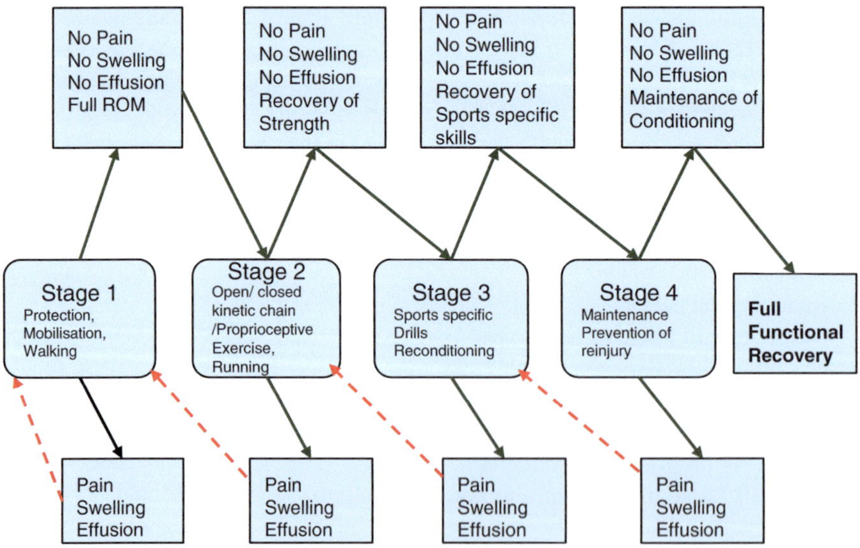

Fig. 3.1 Stages of sport rehabilitation: Adopted from [3]

3.1 Goal-Oriented Rehabilitation Pathway

The three theoretical approaches applied for adherence to sports rehabilitation are as follows [4].

1. Protection Motivation Theory
2. Personal Investment Theory
3. Cognitive Appraisal Model

Protection Motivation Theory helps in predicting adherence to behavior. Athletes adhere to sports injury treatment when they perceive health threats as high, rehabilitation programs to be effective and when they are able to complete their rehabilitation program. This theory does not account for habitual behaviors and social and environmental factors.

According to Personal investment theory, the meaning of the rehabilitation process is determined by the individual characteristics and situational factors. It depends upon the subjective interpretation of meaning which influences personal investment and behavior. The meaning of the injury rehabilitation process can influence adherence to a rehabilitation program.

Cognitive appraisal models suggest that an athlete's behavioral response to a sports injury is influenced by both primary and secondary appraisal processes. Primary appraisal concerned the impact of injury in athletes well-being and goals. Secondary appraisal concerned with the resources of athletes to cope up with the injury. The post-injury behavior of athletes is influenced by emotional responses that arise due to personal and situational factors. The sports medicine/injury practitioner's expectations about an athlete's recovery is also a factor in athletes' compliance to sports injury rehabilitation, as they can influence an athlete's cognitive and emotional responses to their injury. There is a central role for cognitive appraisal models in determining athletes' interpretation of their injuries and adherence to rehabilitation programs.

The sports injury rehabilitation programs should be designed for each patient depending on their individual characteristics, which takes into account the athletes' cognitive, emotional, and behavioral issues.

Key Points

- A structured rehabilitation program is a cornerstone in early return to sports for athletes sustaining injuries.
- There are 4 stages involved in rehabilitation program.
- Factors other than the pathophysiological process of healing also contribute to the recovery process.
- The three theoretical approaches should be taken into consideration for athletes to adhere to the rehabilitation program.

References

1. Bleakley CM. PRICE needs updating, should we call the POLICE? South African J Sports Med. 2016 Jan 22;25(1)
2. Hudson Z. Rehabilitation and return to play after foot and ankle injuries in athletes. Sports Med Arthrosc Rev. 2009 Sep;17(3):203–7.
3. Roi GS. Return to competition following athletic injury: sports rehabilitation as a whole. Medicina de l'esport: Apunts; 2010 Jan 1.
4. Christakou A, Lavallee D. Rehabilitation from sports injuries: from theory to practice. Perspect Public Health. 2009 May;129(3):120–6.

4 Prolotherapy

The chapter starts with a definition of prolotherapy followed by its historical development. While being mainly practiced in the USA initially, it has been spread to other parts of the world bringing more and more research articles. The possible mechanism of action is described, highlighting the different concentrations of dextrose as the main ingredient. It was proposed that different concentrations might have different effects on the body.

Indications and contraindications, as well as possible adverse reactions, are also specified. High safety profile as one of the main advantages of dextrose prolotherapy is emphasized. It is important to master a proper technique of needle positioning.

4.1 Definition of Prolotherapy

Prolo (an abbreviation of proliferation, which means growth or production of cells by multiplication of parts) is a complementary and alternative medical treatment applied to a variety of musculoskeletal conditions. It is an injection-based therapy where different irritant substances are injected to stimulate a healing process. Better insight into the mechanism of action of prolotherapy ingredients prompt scientists to replace the term prolotherapy with more adequate one "regenerative injection therapy - RIT" or more specifically "the injection of growth factors or growth factor production stimulants to promote regeneration of normal cells and tissue" [1]. However, as the term prolotherapy is internationally recognized, the same will be used in this book. Recently the term prolotherapy has broadened to other regenerative procedures.

S. Trebinjac, M. K. Nair, *Regenerative Injections in Sports Medicine*,
https://doi.org/10.1007/978-981-15-6783-4_4

4.2 History of Prolotherapy

It is difficult to find the exact year of origin for the prolotherapy concept because there are some traces of its use reaching around 100 years ago. However, the practical protocol was formalized in 1930 by American surgeon George Hackett [2]. He coined the term "prolotherapy." Hackett and his student Gustav Hemwall are considered as "fathers" of modern prolotherapy.

Dr. Gustav Hemwall helped in forming the prolotherapy foundation in 1969. The foundation was named "Hackett" prolotherapy foundation in tribute to his teacher Dr. George Hackett. Dr. Hemwall started a charity mission and promotion of prolotherapy by bringing some enthusiastic doctors, like Jeff Patterson and Ross Hauser to Honduras, where they were practicing prolotherapy for free and teaching local physicians the new skills. Dr. Jeff Patterson took over this mission after Dr. Hemwall died in 1998. The foundation was renamed to Hackett-Hemwall Foundation, and after Jeff Patterson died in 2014, it was again renamed to the Hackett-Hemwall-Patterson Foundation.

Despite the long history and tremendous experience of pioneers in prolotherapy, this skill remained unknown outside of the USA for decades. However, in the last 10 to 15 years it gained a lot of popularity and the number of courses, research papers, conferences, and communication through electronic media has been increasing dramatically.

"The arts of healing" as prolotherapy was branded, was gradually moved to Europe, where the Italian prolotherapists led by Dr. Stephen Cavallino started the European School of Prolotherapy, with the aim of teaching their colleagues the technique of prolotherapy. Conferences and "hands-on" practice organized in Italy, Greece, and Turkey attracted the doctors from Europe and the Middle East to join the group and acquired theoretical and practical knowledge and skills. With much less publicity than the platelet-rich plasma and stem cells, prolotherapy showed steady growth in the number of trained practitioners all over the world.

4.3 Prolotherapy: Mechanism of Action

A variety of ingredients including polidocanol, manganese, zinc, human growth hormone, pumice, ozone, glycerin, or phenol were used either in a single form or in combination [2]. However, three frequently used solutions with probably different mechanisms of actions are hypertonic dextrose, phenol-glycerol-glucose (P2G), and cod liver extract morrhuate sodium [3]. Among them, hypertonic dextrose (glucose) is the most commonly used ingredient because of the proven therapeutic effect, lack of allergic reactions, and low price. Commonly it is used in a concentration of 12.5%–25% but concentrations of 5% and 10% were also known in practice [4].

The mechanism of action of hypertonic dextrose remains elusive. It is postulated that injection will cause mechanical stress and trigger inflammatory reactions stimulating natural healing cascade. The process is similar to wound healing.

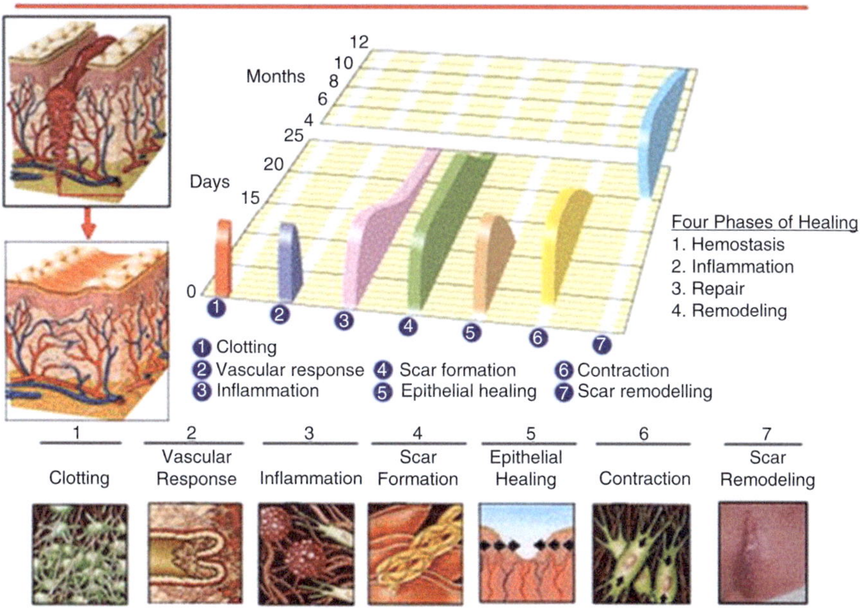

Fig. 4.1 Different stages of wound healing from [6] with permission

Physiological healing of the wound includes inflammatory, proliferative, and remodeling stages. The process ends up with the formation of collagen, which leads to the strengthening of connective tissue and joint stability [5, 6] (Fig. 4.1). It relieves pain and improves the function.

Following this paradigm, the "father" of prolotherapy Dr. George Hackett proposed the cascade of healing model, which includes inflammation, granulation, or proliferation, and maturation [2]. However, the inflammatory response is triggered by different solutions including saline and even needle sticks without any ingredients, so it is not clear what might be the advantage of dextrose [7].

Preclinical studies showed that an increase of dextrose concentration in the cell above 0.1% will stimulate protein and DNA synthesis, cell volume, and proliferation [8]. High glucose concentration has a positive correlation with endothelial cell apoptosis, whereas hyperosmolarity induced endothelial cell necrosis [9].

The interesting hypothesis is that dextrose might initiate internal activation of a variety of growth factors involved in the repair of tendons and ligaments. It was found that different concentrations of dextrose influence the activity of platelet-derived growth factor [10], transforming growth factor-beta (TGFß) [11], heparin-binding epidermal growth factor [12], basic fibroblast growth factor [13], insulin-like growth factor [14], and connective tissue growth factor [15]. It is known that growth factors may play a pro-inflammatory and anti-inflammatory role in the body which correlates with the healing of soft tissues [16]. In animal studies, it was found that the Insulin-like growth factor (IGF 1) improves the collagen structure in the degenerated tendon [17]. Injection of transforming growth factor-beta (TGFß) increases strength and failure load in transected and repaired Achilles tendon [18]. It was confirmed that blocking pro-inflammatory cytokines like IL1 and TNF provides therapeutic effects on Rheumatoid arthritis, Inflammatory Bowel Disease, and Graft Versus Host Disease [19].

It is possible that hyperosmolar dextrose might have dual effects depending on concentration: noninflammatory in low concentration and inflammatory in high concentration. Traditionally used a concentration of 12.5–25% produces an inflammatory response and possible anabolic effect, while a low concentration of 5% might have nerve specific sensory neural mechanisms of pain reduction [7, 20]. Results in vitro confirmed that high concentration of dextrose (12.5% and 15%) cause apoptosis of fibroblasts while low concentration (1%, 5%, and 10%) increase gene expression in angiogenic growth factors (VEGF,PDGFA, PDGFB, and IGF1) and in apoptotic factors (CASP3 and CASP8) in fibroblasts [21].

4.4 Indications and Contraindications for Dextrose Prolotherapy

The joints and soft tissue structures are primary targets of treatment in the field of sports medicine. It includes sports-related injuries but also non-injured conditions like Osgood Schlatter disease for example. The following table shows different anatomical locations, the targeted structures and different concentrations of dextrose injections used for treatment (Table 4.1).

A comprehensive study on adverse reactions related to the treatment of cervical and lumbar spine ligaments concluded that the most common side effect of prolotherapy was pain, followed by stiffness and bruising. Serious complications were not recorded in these studies and among 2000 interventions over a period of 10 years, 69 patients required hospitalization, and 5 patients had permanent nerve damage.

Contraindications and adverse reactions related to dextrose prolotherapy are listed in Table 4.2 [21].

Table 4.1 Anatomical structure treated with dextrose prolotherapy

Location	Targeted structure	Dextrose concentration
Shoulder	Tendons, ligaments, bursas, labrum, periscapular region, capsule, cartilage	<10%,10%, 12.5%, 15%,25%
Elbow	Tendons, ligaments, bursa, capsule, cartilage	<10%,10%,12.5% 15%,25%
Wrist and hand	Tendons, ligaments, capsule, cartilage	<10%,10%, 12.5%, 15%,25%
Hip	Tendons, ligaments, acetabular labrum, Cartilage	<10%,10%, 12.5%,15%,25%
Knee	Tendons, ligaments, meniscus, capsule, cartilage	<10%,10%, 12.5%, 15%,25%
Ankle and foot	Tendons, ligaments. bursa, plantar aponeurosis, capsule cartilage	<10%,10%, 12.5%, 15%,25%
Cervical, thoracic, and lumbosacral spine	Tendons, ligaments, capsule, facet joints, sacroiliac joints, caudal space	<10%,10%, 12.5%, 15%,25%

Table 4.2 Contraindications and adverse reactions related to dextrose prolotherapy

Contraindications	Adverse reactions
Metastatic cancer	Pain
Non-musculoskeletal pain	Stiffness
Spinal anatomical defects	Bruising
Systemic inflammation	Pneumothorax
Morbid obesity	Nerve damage
Bleeding disorders	Temporary systemic reactions
Low pain threshold	Hemorrhage
Inability to perform post-treatment exercises	Spinal cord insult
Whole-body pain	Disk injury
Hepatic conditions	
Allergy to ingredients, main lidocaine	

Dextrose itself is considered as a safe substance even if given in the intravenous form.

It is important to mastermind technical skills because adverse reactions are mainly related to the positioning of the needle in the wrong place. Anatomy of the musculoskeletal system, especially the location of nerves and blood vessels are crucial for safe practice. Injection to the spine is usually learned in advanced courses considering the higher risk for unwanted reactions.

Key Points

- Prolotherapy has been practiced for more than 50 years but mainly in the US private clinics. Recently it gained popularity in the rest of the world.
- It is injection-based therapy using different substances to inject damaged tendons, ligaments, muscles, capsules, and joints. The most common ingredient is hyperosmolar dextrose.
- The mechanism of action of dextrose prolotherapy is not clear and probably depends on the concentration of the injected solution.
- The proper selection of patients is very important taking into account proper indications and recognizing contraindications and possible adverse reactions.
- If applied properly dextrose prolotherapy is a very safe therapeutic modality.
- As it is cheap compared to other regenerative treatments, it can be considered as an alternative in patients who cannot afford the other more expensive options.

References

1. Hackett GS, Hemwall GA, Montgomery GA. Ligament and tendon relaxation treated by Prolotherapy. 5th ed. Gustav A. Hemwall: Oak Park, IL; 1993.
2. Rabago D, Slattengren Andrew DO, Zgierska A. Prolotherapy in primary care practice. Prim Care. 2010;37(1):65–80.
3. Distel LM, Best TM. Prolotherapy: a clinical review of its role in treating chronic musculoskeletal pain. PM R. 2011;3(6 suppl 1):S78–81.

4. DeChellis DM, Cortazzo MH. Regenerative medicine in the field of pain medicine: prolotherapy, platelet-rich plasma therapy, and stem cell therapy-theory and evidence. Tech Reg Anesth Pain Manag. 2011;15(2):74–80.
5. Alexander S, Carlson JW, Schultz Gregory S, Davis Thomas A, Elster Eric A. Topical advances in wound care. Gynecol Oncol. 2008;111(2):S70–80.
6. Jensen KT, Rabago DP, Best TM, Patterson JJ, Vanderby R. Early inflammatory response of knee ligaments to prolotherapy in a rat model. J Orthop Res. 2008 Jun;26(6):816–23.
7. Natarajan R, Gonzales N, Xu L, Nadler JL. Vascular smooth muscle cells exhibit increased growth in response to elevated glucose. Biochem Biophys Res Commun. 1992;187(1):552–60.
8. McGinn S, Poronnik P, King M, Gallery EDM, Pollock CA. High glucose and endothelial cell growth: novel effects independent of autocrine TGF-beta 1 and hyperosmolarity. AJP – Cell Physiology. 2003 Jun 1;284(6):C1374.
9. Di Paloa S, et al. High glucose concentration induces the overexpression of transforming growth factor-beta through the activation of a platelet-derived growth factor loop in human mesangial cells. Am J Pathol. 1996;149:2095–106.
10. Oh J, et al. Sequential effects of high glucose on mesangial cell transforming growth factor-beta 1 and fibronectin synthesis. Kidney Int. 1998;54:1872–8.
11. Fukuda K, et al. High concentration of glucose increases mitogenic responsiveness to heparin-binding epidermal growth factor-like growth factor in rat vascular smooth muscle cells. Arteriosclerosis Thombosis and Vasculature Biology. 1997;17:1962–8.
12. Ohgi S, et al. Glucose modulates growth of gingival fibroblasts and periodontal ligament cells: correlation with expression of basic fibroblast growth factor. J Periodontal Res. 1996;31:579–88.
13. Pugliese G, et al. Increased activity of the insulin-like growth factor system in mesangial cells cultured in high glucose conditions. Relation to glucose-enhanced extracellular matrix production. Diabetologia. 1996;39:775–84.
14. Reeves K. Prolotherapy: injection of growth factors or growth factor production stimulants to growth normal cells or tissue. In: Waldman SD, editor. Pain Management. Philadelphia: Elsevier; 2006. p. 1106–27.
15. Ryabov VV, Kirgizova MA, Suslova TE, Karas SI, Markov VA, Karpov RS. Relationships of growth factors, proinflammatory cytokines, and anti-inflammatory cytokines with long-term clinical results of autologous bone marrow mononuclear cell transplantation in STEMI. PLoS One. 2017;12(5):e0176900.
16. Dahlgren LA, der Meulen V, Marjolein CH, JEA B, Starrak GS, Nixon AJ. Insulin-like growth factor-I improves cellular and molecular aspects of healing in a collagenase-induced model of flexor tendinitis. J Orthop Res. 2002;20(5):910–9.
17. Kashiwagi K, Mochizuki Y, Yasunaga Y, Ishida O, Deie M, Ochi M. Effects of transforming growth factor-β 1 on the early stages of healing of the Achilles tendon in a rat model. Scand J Plast Reconstr Surg Hand Surg. 2004;38(4):193–7.
18. Dinarello CA. Proinflammatory Cytokines. Chest. 2000 Aug;118(2):503–8.
19. Jensen KT, Rabago D, Best TM, et al. Longer term response of knee ligaments to prolotherapy in a rat injury model. Am J Sports Med. 2008;36:1347–57. Crossref, Medline, Google Scholar
20. Güran Ş, Çoban ZD, Karasimav Ö, Demirhan S, Karaağaç N, Örsçelik A, et al. Dextrose solution used for prolotherapy decreases cell viability and increases gene expressions of angiogenic and apopitotic factors. Gulhane Medical Journal. 2018;60(2):42.
21. Dagenais S, Ogunseitan O, Haldeman S, Wooley JR, Newcomb RL. Side effects and adverse events related to Intraligamentous injection of Sclerosing solutions (Prolotherapy) for Back and neck pain: a survey of practitioners. Arch Phys Med Rehabil. 2006;87(7):909–13.

Dextrose Prolotherapy: Preparation Methods and Protocols of Treatment

5

This chapter explains how to prepare the ingredients for prolotherapy and how to apply them. The effective outcome depends on the proper diagnosis and appropriate selection of patients. Diagnosis is not relied on radiological images but rather on specific palpation techniques. The list of ingredients with their concentration is specified. The points, as a possible source of pain, should be marked and injected. Because of this reason, it is different from other regenerative injections procedures like platelet-rich plasma or stem cells. The preparation methods for intra-articular or extra-articular applications are also specified. The original protocol suggested by Hackett and Hemwall related to the number and frequency of procedures is also described. The chapter ends with the results of prolotherapy on animals.

Before starting the prolotherapy procedure, the correct diagnosis must be confirmed. A detailed history of the disease and clinical examination are mandatory before proceeding to laboratory and radiological examination if needed. It is very important to know that prolotherapists will not rely on imaging only, because many times pathology seen on magnetic resonance, for example, is not the primary source of pain. The palpation technique and marking the tender points are actually the most important diagnostic tool before starting injections.

Contraindications to prolotherapy need to be explored as well as potential allergy reactions to prolo ingredients. Allergic reactions are very rare with dextrose injections and may be mainly related to Lidocaine.

The following is the list of items needed for dextrose prolotherapy (Fig. 5.1):

I. 50% dextrose solution
II. 1% or 2% lidocaine solution
III. 0.9% sodium chloride solution
IV. Chlorhexidine gluconate solution
V. Syringes 10 cc, 5 ccs, and 2 ccs
VI. Needles: 27G 1 1/2″, 1 1/4″ and 27G 1″ 25G 2″ 22G/21G 2 3/4″*
VII. Sterile gloves
VIII. Gauze pads, cotton, adhesive bandages

S. Trebinjac, M. K. Nair, *Regenerative Injections in Sports Medicine*,
https://doi.org/10.1007/978-981-15-6783-4_5

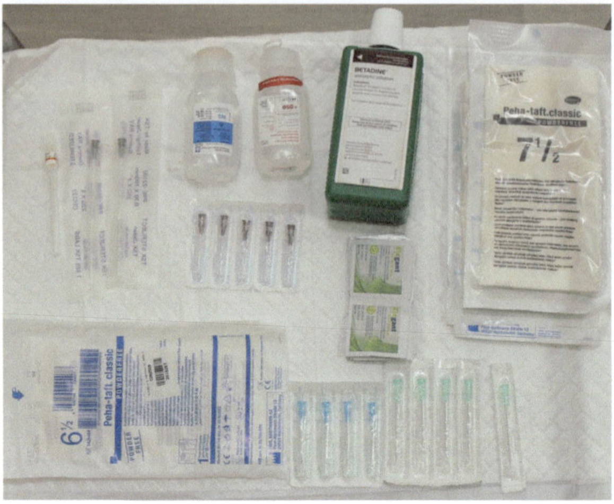

Fig. 5.1 The items needed for dextrose prolotherapy * *The size of the needles depends on the injected area, as deeper structures need longer needles*

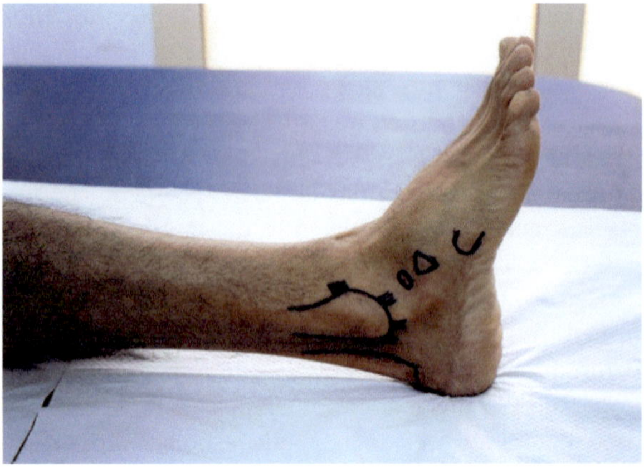

Fig. 5.2 Ankle: Markings on lateral aspect of the joint. Image Courtesy Mr. Glendale Alkuino

The preparation for the prolotherapy procedure starts with palpation of anatomical structures that might be potential sources of pain. Most of the time they are localized at the attachment of tendons and ligaments to the bone. These points are marked with a sterile marker. Here is the example of marking and needle positioning of ankle–foot joint ligaments and tendons (Figs. 5.2, 5.3, 5.4, 5.5, 5.6, 5.7, 5.8, 5.9, and 5.10), but actually each peripheral joint, as well as cervical, thoracic, and lumbosacral spine, have their own specific points to be marked and injected.

Marking points and positioning of the needle for prolotherapy injections—an example of ankle–foot joints, ligaments, and tendons (Figs. 5.2, 5.3, 5.4, 5.5, 5.6, 5.7, 5.8, 5.9, and 5.10).

After the marking points, the whole treated area is sanitized with a disinfectant solution, usually, Chlorhexidine gluconate which seems to be more efficient than Povidone Iodine [1]. The sterilization principles for surgical procedures should be applied, including no-touch technique and wearing sterile gloves.

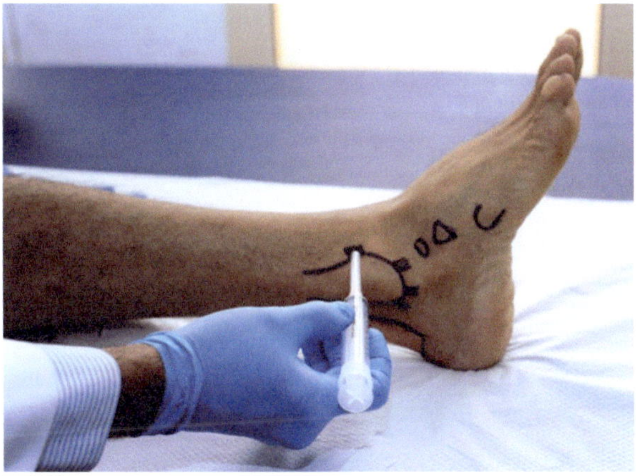

Fig. 5.3 Anterior tibiofibular ligament—different positioning of the needle. Image Courtesy Mr. Glendale Alkuino

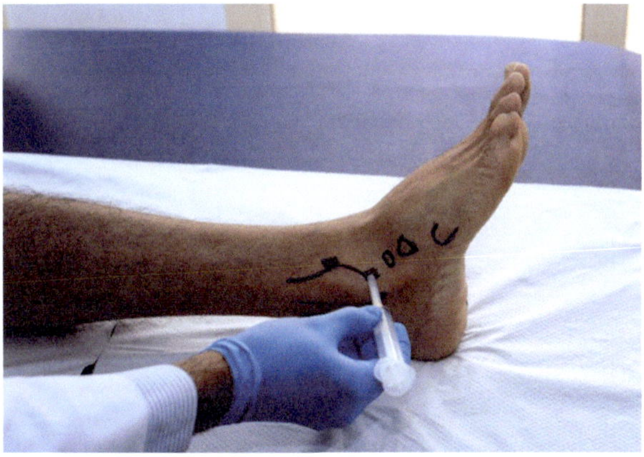

Fig. 5.4 Anterior talofibular ligament (ATFL)—different positioning of the needle. Image Courtesy Mr. Glendale Alkuino

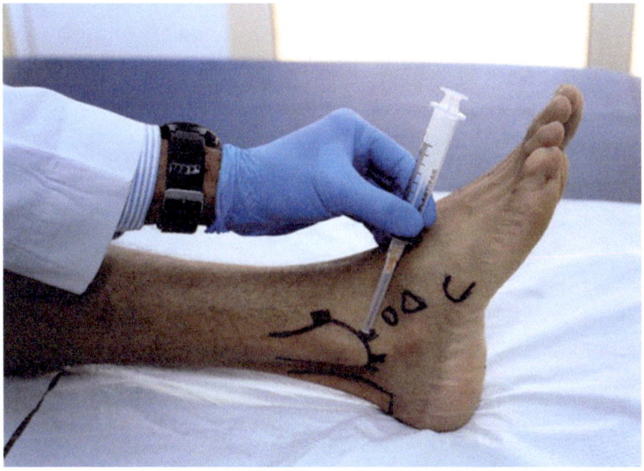

Fig. 5.5 Anterior talofibular ligament (ATFL)—different positioning of the needle. Image Courtesy Mr. Glendale Alkuino

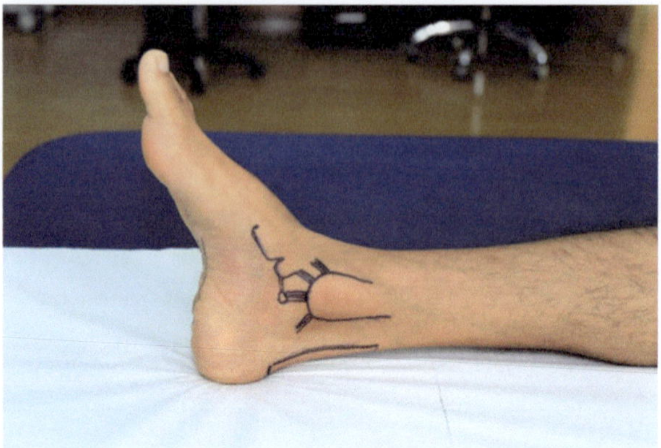

Fig. 5.6 Ankle: Markings on medial aspect of the joint. Image Courtesy Mr. Glendale Alkuino

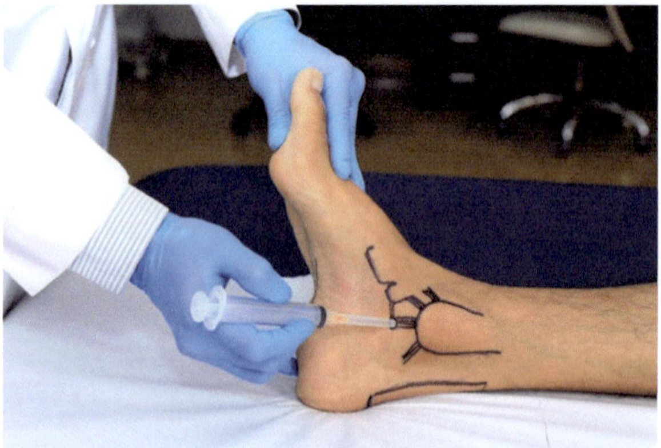

Fig. 5.7 Tibiocalcaneal ligament—different positioning of the needle. Image Courtesy Mr. Glendale Alkuino

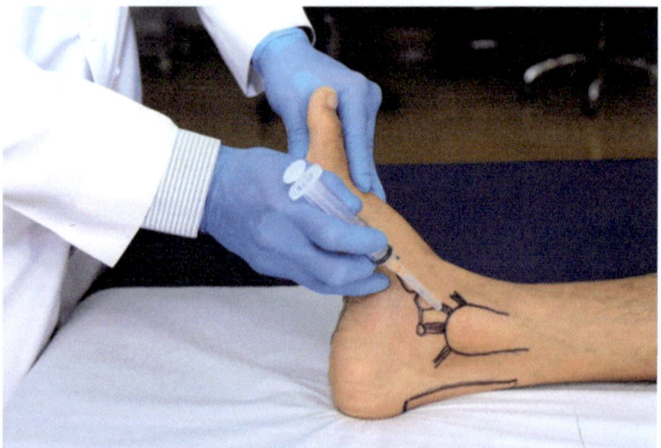

Fig. 5.8 Tibionavicular ligament. Image Courtesy Mr. Glendale Alkuino

After disinfection, local subcutaneous infiltration with a small solution of 1% Lidocaine is done into each marked point. After a local anesthetic is settled down, 50% dextrose mixed with lidocaine and sodium chloride is applied to periarticular

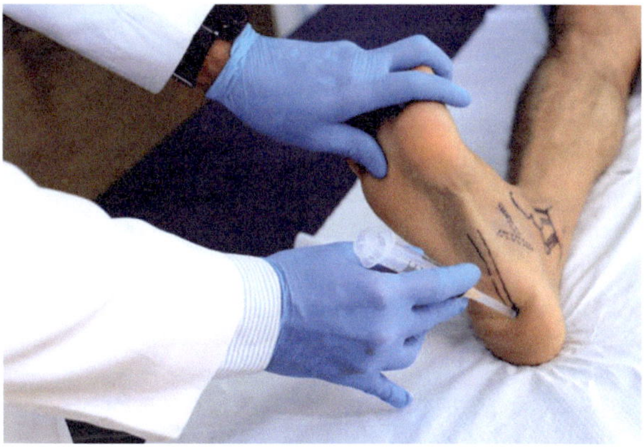

Fig. 5.9 Plantar aponeurosis injection. Image Courtesy Mr. Glendale Alkuino

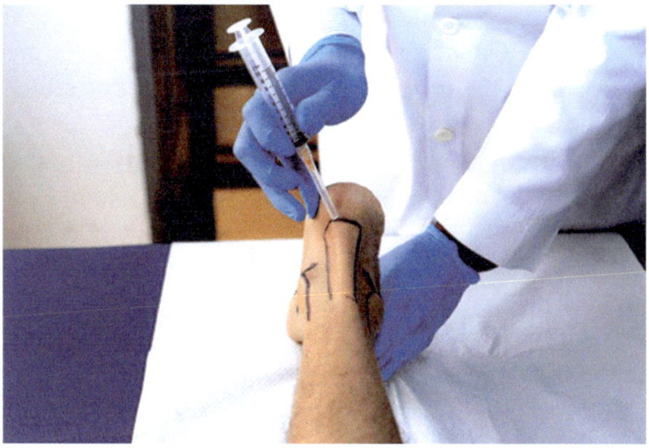

Fig. 5.10 Insertion of the Achilles tendon—positioning of the needle. Image Courtesy Mr. Glendale Alkuino

Table 5.1 The concentration of dextrose prolotherapy solution for Intra-articular and periarticular injections

Intra-articular injections	Concentration	Periarticular injection	Concentration
10 cc syringe: 5 ml—50% dextrose 5 ml—lidocaine 1%	25% dextrose	*10 cc syringe:* 3 ml— 50% dextrose 3 ml—lidocaine 1% 4 ml—0.9 sodium chloride	15% dextrose
		10 cc syringe: 2.5 ml—50% dextrose 5 ml—lidocaine 1% 2.5 ml—o.9% sodium chloride	12.5% dextrose

space. For intra-articular injection, dextrose is mixed with lidocaine but without sodium chloride. Proper technique includes an appropriate angle of needle and depth of penetration. A needle must be placed deep enough to touch the junction of the tendon or ligament to the bone. Different quantities of ingredients are prepared in a 10 cc syringe to get 12.5% or 15% dextrose for periarticular injections and 25% for intra-articular (Table 5.1).

Although the scientific-based protocol is not established, according to the recommendation from the Hackett-Hemwall-Patterson foundation, the procedure has to be repeated five–six times every 4 to 6 weeks apart. Some prolo practitioners reduce the time span between procedures to 2 or 3 weeks and modify the number of sessions according to the condition of the patient. The treatment can be completed in less than five sessions if the patient achieves a resolution of pain but if there is no adequate response after five–six sessions the number can be increased. There are no studies to confirm that either of these different approaches is superior to the other one.

5.1 Animals Study on Dextrose Prolotherapy

A historical article published in 1983 revealed that repeated injections of proliferative substance to the medial collateral ligament of rabbits significantly increased strength, size, and thickness at the bone–ligament junction [2]. This was the first experimental evidence to confirm the therapeutic effect of the sclerosing solution on soft tissue structures.

However, since that time there were only a few animal studies related to the effects of dextrose on the musculoskeletal system. One of them is the study investigating the effect of 15% Dextrose on the medial collateral ligament of the rats. The study confirmed that the cross-sectional area of the ligament was significantly enlarged compared with no injections or saline injections as a control group, but ligament laxity was not altered by dextrose injections [3]. In mice with contusion induced muscle injury, dextrose prolotherapy showed better muscle recovery than saline and NSAID. It was presented by suppression of macrophage response (F4/80 protein decreased), muscle satellite cell regeneration (desmin protein increased), improving muscle damage (decrease in LDH and CK). They found that 10% of dextrose showed a better therapeutic effect on the recovery of muscle contusion than 20% or 30% dextrose and diclofenac as a nonsteroidal anti-inflammatory drug [4]. In another study on rabbits carpal tunnel syndrome, it was found that energy absorption in sub synovial connective tissue (SSCT) and stiffness in the carpal tunnel region is increased after double injection of 10% dextrose compared to saline. At the same time, there were no changes in the nerve conduction study. This model may be helpful to study the effect of synovial fibrosis on the development of carpal tunnel syndrome (CTS) [5].

Key Points

- Preparation of dextrose prolotherapy to get appropriate concentration and skilled injection technique are two major elements of successful treatment.
- Palpation as a part of clinical examination is more important than radiographic findings.
- Application of dextrose injections is different from other therapies because it includes all damaged structures inside and around joints as a potential source of pain.

- There is no unified treatment protocol but there is a recommendation by the founder of prolotherapy based on their personal experience.
- A limited number of animal studies provided promising results.

References

1. Firas A, Michael Q, Ronan C, Arnold H. Chlorhexidine-alcohol versus povidone-iodine for pre-operative skin preparation: a systematic review and meta-analysis. Int J Surg Open. 2015;1:41–6.
2. Liu YK, Tipton CM, Matches RD, Bedford TG, Maynard JA, Walmer HC. An in situ study of a Sclerosing solution in rabbit medial collateral ligaments and its junction strength. Connect Tissue Res. 1983;11(2–3):95–102.
3. Kristina T, Jensen David P, Rabago Thomas M, Best Jeffrey J, Patterson Ray Vanderby J. Response of knee ligaments to Prolotherapy in a rat injury model. Am J Sports Med. 2008 Jul 1;36(7):1347–57.
4. Tsai S, Hsu Y, Lee M, Huang H, Huang C, Tung Y. Effects of dextrose prolotherapy on contusion-induced muscle injuries in mice. Int J Med Sci. 2018;15(11):1251–9.
5. Yoshii Y, Zhao C, Schmelzer JD, Low PA, An K, Amadio PC. Effects of hypertonic dextrose injections in the rabbit carpal tunnel. J Orthop Res. 2011 Jul;29(7):1022–7.

6 Clinical Applications of Dextrose Prolotherapy in Sports

Prolotherapy is applied in a form of injections to tendons, ligaments, muscles, capsules, and joints. It can provide benefits to patients suffering shoulder, elbow, wrist/hand, hip, knee, and ankle/foot pain. Neck and back injuries are also treated with prolotherapy. This chapter explains in detail what are the most common sports injuries affecting peripheral joints, the mechanism of their onset, and how dextrose prolotherapy can help in their management.

Scientific papers related to the application of dextrose injections to a variety of conditions are listed in the form of tables. Conclusions and recommendations from each study are highlighted. More randomized controlled clinical trials are recommended.

6.1 Shoulder

The treatment of shoulder injuries is either conservative or surgical. The choice depends not only on the type of injury but also on patient age, comorbidities, and preferred style of life. The majority of mild and moderate injuries can be treated with rest, physical and manual therapy, nonsteroidal anti-inflammatory medications, and corticosteroid injections. Surgery is reserved for more complicated cases and includes both arthroscopic and open surgery. Postoperative rehabilitation is an integrative part of treatment.

Several studies related to the treatment of shoulder pathology with dextrose prolotherapy were published in the last 10 years. They include noncontrolled [1–3], as well as controlled trials [4–8]. There is a lot of heterogeneity between these studies in terms of dextrose concentration and treatment frequency. Also, targeted structures are different. Study design ranges from case reports to blind randomized control trials (Tables 6.1 and 6.2).

The overall results show that dextrose prolotherapy is an effective treatment of pain reduction and functional improvement. Significant adverse events were not

S. Trebinjac, M. K. Nair, *Regenerative Injections in Sports Medicine*,
https://doi.org/10.1007/978-981-15-6783-4_6

Table 6.1 Dextrose prolotherapy for shoulder pathology; noncontrolled studies

Authors	Title	Injected structure	Study design	Dextrose concentration	Number of sessions	Results	Conclusion
Seenauth C.et al.	Dextrose prolotherapy for chronic shoulder pain: A case report.	GH* joint space, the AC* joint, the subacromial space, and the insertion of the supraspinatus.	Case record study	Mean 22.8%	3 sessions	Pain reduction of 90%. Complete functional improvement	The dextrose prolotherapy may be an effective alternative to surgery for chronic shoulder pain.
Trebinjac S. et al.	Long-term effect of prolotherapy on symptomatic rotator cuff tendinopathy.	Rotator cuff tendons, AC, and GH joints	Retrospective case record study	15% periarticular and 25% intra-articular	6	Significant pain reduction and functional improvement from baseline. 85.71% would recommend prolotherapy	Hyperosmolar dextrose prolotherapy may result in a significant reduction of pain and disability index in adult patients with chronic rotator cuff tendinopathy, without eliciting long-lasting side effects.
Hsieh P. et al.	Ultrasound-guided prolotherapy for acromial enthesopathy and acromioclavicular joint arthropathy: single-arm prospective study	Acromial enthesopathy and acromioclavicular joint	Prospective single-arm study	15%	2 sessions	20 of 31 patients reported substantial pain reduction	Acromial enthesopathy and acromioclavicular joint arthropathy could be successfully treated with the US* guided 15% dextrose.

Abbreviations: **GH* Glenohumeral joint, **AC*: Acromioclavicular joint, **US* Ultrasound

Table 6.2 Dextrose prolotherapy for shoulder pathology: controlled studies

Authors	Title	Injected structure	Study design	Dextrose concentration	Number of sessions	Results	Conclusion
Seven MM et al.	Effectiveness of Prolotherapy in the treatment of chronic rotator cuff lesions.	Rotator cuff tendon + deltoid, pectoralis minor, biceps brachii, and coracobrachialis. Inferior GH ligament	RCT* dextrose versus physiotherapy	15%	2-6., mean 5.23	Significant improvement in pain score and shoulder function in prolotherapy compared to PT* group.	The dextrose prolotherapy is a safe and efficient therapeutic option for the rotator cuff lesions.
Bertrand H et al.	Dextrose Prolotherapy versus control injections in painful rotator cuff tendinopathy.	Rotator cuff tendons	RCT-dextrose versus saline	25%	3	Superior long-term pain improvement and patient satisfaction in the dextrose group	The result cannot be attributed to the regenerative effect
Lee, doo-Hyung et al.	Prolotherapy for refractory rotator cuff disease: a retrospective case-control study of 1-year follow-up.	Rotator cuff tendons	Retrospective case-control study, dextrose versus conservative treatment (NSAID* and PT*)	16.5%	Average 4.8+/−1.3	Improvement in pain, disability, isometric strength and AROM* in dextrose group	Limitation of the study: Non-randomized, retrospective trial
Lin C et al.	Effects of hypertonic dextrose injection on chronic supraspinatus tendinopathy of the shoulder: a randomized placebo-controlled trial.	Supraspinatus tendon	RCT placebo controlled	20%	1	Improvement in pain reduction and function after 2 weeks in favor of dextrose prolo, but not after 6 weeks	Dextrose prolotherapy reduces pain, disability, and AROM in a short period of time.
George J. et al.	Comparative effectiveness of ultrasound-guided Intratendinous Prolotherapy injection with conventional treatment to treat focal supraspinatus tendinosis.	Supraspinatus tendon	RCT dextrose prolotherapy versus PT	12.5%	1	Shoulder abduction and sleep scores significantly improved in the prolotherapy group. The echogenicity of the injured area significantly increased.	This is a small sample study confirming the efficacy of US-guided dextrose prolotherapy on shoulder abduction and sleeping quality. The change in echogenicity was also documented by the US.

Abbreviations: **RCT* Randomized control trial,**PT* Physical therapy **NSAID*: Nonsteroidal anti-inflammatory drugs, **AROM* Active range of motion

reported in any of the above studies. As the treated patients were not exclusively belonging to athletics, the results cannot be extrapolated to this category, so we cannot assume the same results in sports injuries. However, considering the same pathology among sportspeople, we infer at least similar or even better results to be expected as there are fewer comorbidities, a strong immune system, and better motivation for recovery in sportspeople.

6.2 Elbow

Elbow injuries are common among athletes. Due to chronicity in the majority of cases, they are difficult to treat. Oral NSAIDs have a very limited effect considering the lack of inflammation. However, they are frequently prescribed together with physiotherapy. Surgery is reserved for difficult conditions resistant to conservative therapy.

The most frequent prolotherapy research is related to lateral epicondylitis [9, 10]. In double-blinded RCT prolotherapy was compared with corticosteroid injections. In this study, dextrose was mixed with P2g (phenol–glycerin–glucose) and morrhuate sodium (extract of cod liver oil), so it is not clear whether dextrose alone provided benefit or it is due to the effect of other components. In both groups, significant improvement was achieved from the baseline, without difference between groups after 3 and 6 months [11]. Recently published single-blinded study comparing dextrose prolotherapy with physiotherapy used separately or in combination showed no difference between these two modalities. However, all groups showed significant improvement from the baseline 52 weeks after the treatment [12].

The case series study on nonspecific elbow pain treated with dextrose prolotherapy confirmed that more than 90% of patients get pain relief. We could find only one study mentioning morphological changes before and after dextrose prolotherapy in lateral epicondylitis [13]. (Table 6.3).

We were not able to identify studies investigating dextrose prolotherapy for the treatment of medial epicondylitis, triceps tendinopathy, or any of elbow ligaments.

Like in any other peripheral joint injections, positioning of the needle is very important while injecting around the elbow because of the proximity of the blood vessels (cubital artery and vein) and nerves (radial and ulnar nerves). Overall, adverse reactions and side effects are uncommon, and treating the elbow joint with dextrose injections is considered a safe procedure.

6.3 Wrist and Hand

Standardized treatment of wrist and hand injuries includes immobilization and pain management in the acute stage, followed by physical therapy and surgery when needed. Scaphoid bone fracture and triangular fibrocartilaginous complex injury are difficult to treat and usually need long-term rehabilitation.

Table 6.3 Dextrose prolotherapy for elbow pathology

Authors	Title	Injected structure	Study design	Dextrose concentration	Number of sessions	Results	Conclusion
Rabago et al.	Prolotherapy in primary health care practice	Tendons of lateral epicondyle	RCT* Dextrose versus saline	(1 part 5% sodium morrhuate, 1.5 parts 50% dextrose, 0.5 parts 4% lidocaine, 0.5 parts 0.5% sensorcaine and 3.5 parts normal saline Control group: normal saline	3	Significantly decrease pain and increase isometric strength in dextrose/morrhuate group Improved grip strength from the based line	Dextrose/ morrhuate was well tolerated. Promising results need to be confirmed in RCT studies
Yelland et al.	Prolotherapy injections and physiotherapy used singly and in combination for lateral epicondylalgia: a single-blinded randomized clinical trial	Lateral epicondyle	Single-blinded RCT	20% dextrose	4	Significant improvement from baseline in each separate group and in combination after 52 weeks, There was no significant difference between groups.	Prolotherapy was not better than physiotherapy neither as a separate nor in combination after 12 month of trial.
Shin et al.	The effect of Prolotherapy on lateral epicondylitis of elbow.	Tendons of lateral epicondyle	Case series	15% dextrose	3	Significant pain reduction, more present in patients without tendon tear	Prolotherapy is an effective treatment for lateral epicondylitis. US* can be a useful diagnostic method to predict the effect of prolotherapy.
Carayannopoulos et al.	Prolotherapy versus corticosteroid injections for the treatment of lateral epicondylitis: A randomized controlled trial	Tendon of lateral epicondyle	RCT double-blinded.	Dextrose 12.5% + P2G* + Morrhuate sodium combination with	2	Significant improvement from the baseline in both groups. No difference between groups after 3 and 6 months	Prolotherapy can be considered as a safe and efficient treatment for lateral epicondylitis.
Park et al.	Ultrasonographic findings on healing of torn tendon in patients with lateral epicondylitis after prolotherapy	Lateral epicondyle	Case series	15% dextrose	2 to 6 injections	VAS* reduction, changes in echogenicity and fibrillar pattern after prolotherapy	There is confirmation of the healing of torn tendon after the application of dextrose prolotherapy.

Abbreviations: **RCT* Randomized control trial, ** P2G* Phenol- Glycerin-Glucose,**US* Ultrasound,**VAS* Visual analog scale

Prolotherapy is commonly used for wrist pain [14], but there are only a few studies investigating its efficacy. In a randomized controlled trial, the efficacy of dextrose prolotherapy injections in peri scaphoid and peri lunate ligaments with lidocaine showed no significant difference in grip strength and range of motion [15]. In another retrospective case series study treatment of wrist joints with dextrose prolotherapy reduced pain, increased range of motion, reduced anxiety, depression, and use of medications. Dextrose prolotherapy in osteoarthritis of the hand found significantly improved pain and movement of fingers and thumb flexion and nonsignificant effect on pain at rest and with grip [16]. In another RCT dextrose, prolotherapy showed a better long-term effect than corticosteroid injections in the treatment of the first carpometacarpal joint [17]. (Table 6.4).

6.4 Hip and Groin

Dextrose prolotherapy was used for the treatment of osteitis pubis and adductor tendinopathy in elite male kicking sports athletes [18]. A similar study presented a positive effect of dextrose prolotherapy on elite athletes who failed other conservative treatments [19]. (Table 6.5).

We were not able to identify studies related to dextrose injections to other hip structures and also there were no randomized controlled trials comparing dextrose prolotherapy with placebo or other modalities.

6.5 Knee

Like with other joint injuries different types of conservative therapy are prescribed. The most common is rest and ice in the acute stage followed by nonsteroidal anti-inflammatory medications and physical therapy. In addition, injection treatments with corticosteroids, hyaluronic acid, platelet-rich plasma are frequently applied. Recently, mesenchymal stem cell therapy gained momentum in the management of knee osteoarthritis. Surgery is usually indicated for complete anterior cruciate ligament tear and grade 3 and 4 meniscus tear.

Dextrose prolotherapy is frequently used in the management of knee injuries and degenerative changes. The largest number of studies on the prolotherapy treatment was associated with knee joints. They are basically related to knee osteoarthritis and not specifically targeting the sports population. Both uncontrolled and controlled studies confirmed the efficacy and safety of prolotherapy [20–23]. Tables 6.6 and 6.7 several systematic reviews with and without meta-analysis also concluded that dextrose prolotherapy is an efficient and safe option for the management of knee osteoarthritis [24, 25] and Osgood Schlatter disease [26] (Table 6.8). Results of uncontrolled, controlled and systematic review studies are presented in tables 6.6, 6.7 and 6.8.

Despite a relatively large number of studies, a lack of evidence related to particular sports injuries, like ACL and meniscus tear makes dextrose prolotherapy research very limited and unspecific for sports cohort. However, considering that

Table 6.4 Dextrose prolotherapy for wrist and hand pathology

Authors	Title	Injected structure	Study design	Dextrose concentration	Number of sessions	Results	Conclusion
Hooper R. et al.	Randomized controlled trial for the treatment of chronic dorsal wrist pain with dextrose prolotherapy.	Peri scaphoid, and peril lunate ligaments,	RCT* lidocaine (placebo) versus lidocaine/dextrose	20%	6	In dextrose lidocaine group strength and ROM* significantly improved but did not reach MCID*	Efficacy of dextrose prolotherapy comparing with lidocaine (placebo) was not confirmed.
Hauser R. et al.	Dextrose Prolotherapy for unresolved wrist pain	Wrist joints-tendons and ligaments	Retrospective case series	15%	Average of 3.6	Reduced pain, increased ROM, reduced anxiety, depression and use of medications	Dextrose prolotherapy might be an efficient and safe therapeutic option for the management of wrist and hand injuries.
Reeves KD, Hassanein K.	Randomized, prospective, placebo-controlled double-blind study of dextrose Prolotherapy for osteoarthritis thumb and finger (DIP*, PIP*, and trapeziometacarpal) joints: evidence of clinical efficacy	Medial and lateral aspects of each affected joint	RCT	10%	3	Pain with movements of fingers and flexion ROM improved significantly in the dextrose group.	Dextrose prolotherapy is efficient in the treatment of pain and ROM in patients with finger osteoarthritis.
Jahangiri et al.	Hypertonic dextrose versus corticosteroid local injection for the treatment of osteoarthritis in the first carpometacarpal joint: a double-blind randomized clinical trial	First carpometacarpal joint	Dextrose prolotherapy versus corticosteroid (methylprednisolone acetate)	20%	3	At 1 month better outcome with corticosteroid and after 6 months with dextrose prolotherapy	Long-term effects of dextrose prolotherapy are more favorable than the effects of corticosteroid injection for the treatment of first carpometacarpal joint.

Abbreviations: **RCT* Randomized controlled trials,**ROM* Range of motion,**MCID* Minimal clinically important difference,**DIP* Distal interphalangeal, **PIP* Proximal interphalangeal

Table 6.5 Dextrose prolotherapy for hip and groin pathology

Authors	Title	Injected structure	Study design	Dextrose concentration	Number of sessions	Results	Conclusion
Topol GA et al.	Efficacy of dextrose prolotherapy in elite male kicking-sport athletes with chronic groin pain.	Thigh adductor origins, suprapubic abdominal insertions, and symphysis pubis	Consecutive case series	12.5%	2.8 average	20 out of 24 patients were pain-free and 22 out of 24 resumed sports activities without restrictions	Dextrose prolotherapy is efficient in reduction of groin pain in elite rugby and soccer players.
Topol GA and Reeves KD	Regenerative injection of elite athletes with career-altering chronic groin pain who fails conservative treatment: a consecutive case series	Abdominal and adductor attachments on the pubis	Consecutive case series	12.5%	3 average	VAS* pain reduction in 82%, Niershe scale improvement 78%, 66 out of 75 returned to unrestricted sports	Athletes return to full elite performance after injection of dextrose prolotherapy

Abbreviation; **VAS* Visual analog scale

Table 6.6 Dextrose prolotherapy for knee osteoarthritis (uncontrolled studies)

Authors	Title	Injected structure	Study design	Dextrose concentration	Number of sessions	Results	Conclusion
Eslamian F. and Amouzandeh B	Therapeutic effects of prolotherapy with intra-articular dextrose injection in patients with moderate knee osteoarthritis: a single-arm study with 6 month follow-up	Knee joint intra-articular	Single-arm prospective study	20%	3	Significant improvement after 24 weeks in pain, ROM* and WOMAC*	Needs for RCT* s
Reeves KD et al.	Chondrogenic effect of Intraarticular hypertonic dextrose (prolotherapy) in severe knee osteoarthritis	Knee intra-articular	Case series	12.5%	4–6	Cartilage growth, WOMAC* score improved	The possible disease-modifying effects, needs controlled studies.
Rabago et al.	Hypertonic dextrose injections (prolotherapy) for knee osteoarthritis results of a single-arm uncontrolled study with 1-year follow-up.:	Knee joint intra-articular and extra-articular	Post clinical trial open-label follow-up	15% PA* and 25% IA*	3–5	Progressive improvement in WOMAC* and KPS* score.	Dextrose prolotherapy improves pain, function, and stiffness in knee osteoarthritis. It is a safe procedure.

Abbreviations:**ROM* Range of motion, **WOMAC* Western Ontario and McMaster Universities Osteoarthritis Index, *KPS** Knee pain score **RCT* Randomized controlled trials,**I.A* Intraarticular,**P.A* Periarticular

Table 6.7 Dextrose prolotherapy for knee osteoarthritis - Randomized controlled trials

Authors	Title	Injected Structures	Study design	Dextrose concentration	Number of sessions	Results	Conclusions
Rabago et al.	Qualitative assessment of patients receiving prolotherapy for knee osteoarthritis in a multimethod study	Intra-articular and extra-articular injections	A qualitative study using semi-structured in-depth interview	Not mentioned	3–5	Eighty-two percent of participants described decreased knee pain and improved knee function without substantial side effects.	The study provides better insight into the meaning of prolotherapy for patients.
Rezasoltani Z et al.	Periarticular dextrose prolotherapy instead of intra-articular injection for pain and functional improvement in knee osteoarthritis	Periarticular injections	RCT* (double-blind)	10% I.A* and 20% P.A.*	5	VAS* was significantly lower in P.A* than in I.A* group at the 2,3, 4, and5-months visit.	Periarticular injections could be an adequate alternative to intra-articular injections.
Topol GA et al.	Hyperosmolar dextrose injection for recalcitrant Osgood-Schlatter disease	Periarticular injection (apophysis of the tibia and patellar tendon insertion)	RCT (double blind)	12.5% dextrose with and without 1% lidocaine	3 and continue dextrose injections monthly if needed	Asymptomatic sports practicing was more common in dextrose treatment than treatment with lidocaine or usual care	Dextrose injections are safe and superior to usual care in unaltered sport and asymptomatic sport.

Abbreviations: **RCT* Randomized controlled trials,**I.A* Intraarticular,**P.A* Periarticular,**VAS* Visual analog scale

Table 6.8 Dextrose prolotherapy for knee osteoarthritis (systematic reviews)

Authors	Title	Injected Structures	Study design	Dextrose concentration	Number of sessions	Results	Conclusions
Hassan F. et al.	The effectiveness of prolotherapy in treating knee osteoarthritis in adults: a systematic review.	I.A. and P.A knee injections	A systematic review including controlled and uncontrolled studies	10–25%	2–5 with a different time span between sessions	In all studies improvement from the baseline was reported and in 4 studies significant improvement compared to the control group	Moderate evidence suggests that prolotherapy is safe and can help achieve significant symptomatic control in individuals with OA.
Krstičević M. et al.	Proliferative injection therapy for osteoarthritis: a systematic review. International Orthopedics	I.A. and P.A. knee joint injections	A systematic review of RCTs	10–25% dextrose	1–5 with a different time span between injections	Limited evidence from low-quality clinical trials with small numbers of participants indicates that prolotherapy may be effective and safe for the treatment of OA.	Low-quality clinical trials that offer limited evidence supporting the use of proliferative injection therapy in the treatment of osteoarthritis. Those studies do not provide answers about the most effective solution, the optimal frequency of administration or optimal co-interventions.
Sit RW, et al.	Hypertonic dextrose injections (prolotherapy) in the treatment of symptomatic knee osteoarthritis: a systematic review and meta-analysis	I.A. and P.A. knee joint injections	A systematic review and meta-analysis-randomized and quasi-randomized trials	10–25% dextrose	Not reported	Dextrose prolotherapy provide positive effect compared to saline and exercise	The small number of studies and small sample sizes, as well as moderate heterogeneity among the studies limited interpretation of results.

Abbreviations:**ROM* Range of motion, **WOMAC* Western Ontario and McMaster Universities Osteoarthritis Index, *KPS** Knee pain score **RCT* Randomized controlled trials,**I.A* Intraarticular,**P.A* Periarticular,**VAS* Visual analog scale

prolotherapy in its original teaching treats the whole joint, rather than specific anatomical parts, it can be probably more suitable for multiple structures damages rather than isolated parts.

6.6 Ankle and Foot

The majority of ankle and foot injuries are treated conservatively and management is similar to other joint injuries. Pain modulation and functional restoration by physical therapy are the most frequently prescribed therapeutic options.

The possibility of treating ankle pain with prolotherapy was mentioned in Mayo clinic newsletters in 2005 [27]. Since then there have been several published studies in relation to ankle and foot management by dextrose prolotherapy. Hauser and co-authors documented the benefit of prolotherapy for ankle and foot injuries [28]. In another case series study with a small sample size, pain reduction is confirmed by the Visual Analog Scale [29]. A retrospective observational study of the nonspecific ankle and foot pain showed improvement in pain, stiffness, walking ability, anxiety, and depression

. In more specific studies related to the treatment of Achilles tendinopathy, dextrose prolotherapy in combination with eccentric exercise was more efficient than exercise alone or prolotherapy alone [30]. In a pilot study, dextrose injections cause not only pain reduction but also morphological changes after Achilles tendon tear, indicating the healing process [31]. In a single-arm study, a new fibrous tissue at the place of injury was found 28 weeks after the treatment, and pain reduction reached 81% after 14 months [32]. In a condition of chronic plantar fasciitis, PRP and dextrose prolotherapy showed similar results 2 and 6 months after the treatment [33]. Table 6.9 summarizes the details of the publications.

From the above, it is obvious that there is a shortage of high-quality studies comparing dextrose prolotherapy with other treatment modalities commonly used for ankle–foot injuries. Also, like with other prolotherapy publications, there are not enough specific studies related to athletes' cohorts. However, the majority of results published so far are promising and giving a solid foundation for further randomized controlled trials.

Key Points

- The majority of sports injuries are related to soft tissue periarticular structures, bones, and joints.
- Dextrose prolotherapy can be a good solution for chronic injuries located at the shoulder, elbow, wrist/hand, hip, knee, and ankle/foot.
- Different concentrations might be used for different locations of injury, higher concentrations are used for intra-articular injections compared to periarticular.
- There are plenty of clinical studies on humans confirming the efficacy and safety of dextrose prolotherapy applications. However, there are still not enough high-quality randomized control trials. Comparative studies with PRP and mesenchymal stem cells are also missing.

Table 6.9 Dextrose prolotherapy for the ankle and foot

Authors	Title	Injected structures	Study design	Dextrose concentration	Number of sessions	Results	Conclusions
Ross A. Hauser et al.	A systematic review of dextrose prolotherapy for chronic musculoskeletal pain.	Tendons, ligaments, joints, muscles	A systematic review	From 10% –25%	Different in different studies	Overall positive effect on pain reduction and function. In few studies documented morphological changes as a sign of healing of injured tissue	Promising results but there is a lack of high-quality controlled studies
Kim B.	The effect of prolotherapy for chronic pain of the musculoskeletal system.	Ankle joint, nonspecific location	Case record	15%	2 sessions	Pain reduction, measured by VAS* scale	Very small sample, only three patients.
Yelland MJ. et al.	Prolotherapy injections and eccentric loading exercises for painful Achilles tendinosis: a randomized trial.	Achilles tendon	RCT*	20%	4–12	Dextrose prolotherapy in combination with eccentric loading exercise is more efficient than eccentric exercise alone.	A combination of dextrose prolotherapy and eccentric loading exercise might be an efficient treatment for chronic Achilles tendinopathies.
Maxwell NJ. et al.	Sonographically guided Intratendinous injection of hyperosmolar dextrose to treat chronic tendinosis of the Achilles tendon: A pilot study.	Achilles tendon	Pilot study	25%	Average of 4 treatments	Pain reduction at rest 89%, during daily activities 84% and at exercise 78%	Morphology of the tendon was changed indicating the healing process.
Ryan M. et al.	Sonographically guided Intratendinous injection of hyperosmolar dextrose for chronic insertional and mid-portion Achilles tendinosis.	Achilles tendon	Case record	25%	Average of 5 treatments	Pain reduction measured by VAS at rest, during daily activities, and during exercise resulting in an improvement of 31%, 41%, and 50%, respectively, at a 28-month follow-up	Tendon injections to the mid-portion or insertion of the Achilles tendon produce pain reduction maintained for more than 2 years after the treatment.
Lee JH and Kim E.	Autologous platelet-rich plasma versus dextrose prolotherapy for the treatment of chronic recalcitrant plantar fasciitis.	Plantar fascia	Single blinded RCT	15%	2 treatments	Improvement in pain and function in both groups. Similar results after 2 and 6 months	Both, PRP* and dextrose prolotherapy are efficient in the treatment of chronic plantar fasciitis. There is no significant difference between 2 and 6 months.

Abbreviations:**VAS* Visual analog scale, **RCT* Randomized control trial, **PRP* Platelet-rich plasma

References

1. Seenauth C, Inouye V, Langland JO. Dextrose Prolotherapy for chronic shoulder pain: a case report. Altern Ther Health Med. 2018 Jan;24(1):56–60.
2. Trebinjac S, Kitchbi H. Long-term effect of Prolotherapy on symptomatic rotator cuff tendinopathy. J Health Sci. 2015 Dec 15;5(3):93.
3. Hsieh P, Chiou H, Wang H, Lai Y, Lin Y. Ultrasound-guided Prolotherapy for acromial Enthesopathy and Acromioclavicular joint Arthropathy: a single-arm prospective study. J Ultrasound Med. 2018 Aug;31
4. Seven M, Ersen O, Akpancar S, Ozkan H, Turkkan S, Yıldız Y, Koca K. Effectiveness of Prolotherapy in the treatment of chronic rotator cuff lesions. Orthop Traumatol Surg Res. 2017;103(3):427–33.
5. Bertrand H, Reeves KD, Bennett CJ, Bicknell S, Cheng A-L. Dextrose Prolotherapy versus control injections in painful rotator cuff Tendinopathy. Arch Phys Med Rehabil. 2016;97(1):17–25.
6. Lee D-H, Kwack K-S, Rah UW, Yoon S-H. Prolotherapy for refractory rotator cuff disease: retrospective case-control study of 1-year follow-up. Arch Phys Med Rehabil. 2015;96(11):2027–32.
7. Lin C, Huang C, Huang S. Effects of hypertonic dextrose injection on chronic supraspinatus tendinopathy of the shoulder: randomized placebo-controlled trial. Eur J Phys Rehabil Med. 2018 Dec 13;55(4):480–7.
8. George J, Li SC, Jaafar Z, Hamid MSA. Comparative effectiveness of ultrasound-guided Intratendinous Prolotherapy injection with conventional treatment to treat focal supraspinatus Tendinosis. Scientifica. 2018;2018:4384159–7.
9. Rabago D, Slattengren A, Zgierska A. Prolotherapy in primary care practice. Prim Care. 2010;37(1):65–80.
10. Shin J, et al. The effect of Prolotherapy on lateral epicondylitis of the elbow. J Korean Academy of Rehabilitation Med. 2002;26:764–8.
11. Carayannopoulos A, Borg-Stein J, Sokolof J, Meleger A, Rosenberg D. Prolotherapy versus corticosteroid injections for the treatment of lateral Epicondylosis: a randomized controlled trial. PM&R. 2011;3(8):706–15.
12. Yelland M, Rabago D, Ryan M, Ng S, Vithanachchi D, Manickaraj N, et al. Prolotherapy injections and physiotherapy used singly and in combination for lateral epicondylalgia: a single-blinded randomised clinical trial. BMC Musculoskelet Disord. 2019 Nov 3;20(1):509.
13. Park JH, Song IS, Lee JB, et al. Ultrasonographic findings of healing of torn tendon in the patients with lateral epicondylitis after prolotherapy. J Korean Soc Med Ultrasound. 2003;22(3):177–83.
14. Hauser R, et al. Prolo your pain away! 3rd ed. Oak Park, IL: Beulah Land Press; 2007. p. 126–38.
15. Hooper RA, Hildebrand K, Faris P, Westaway M, Freiheit E. Randomized controlled trial for the treatment of chronic dorsal wrist pain with dextrose prolotherapy. Int Musculoskeletal Med. 2011 Sep;33(3):100–6.
16. Reeves K, Hassanein K. Randomized, prospective placebo-controlled double-blind study of dextrose prolotherapy for osteoarthritic thumb and finger joints: evidence of clinical efficacy. J Altern Complement Med. 2000;6(4):311–20.
17. Jahangiri A, Moghaddam FR, Najafi S. Hypertonic dextrose versus corticosteroid local injection for the treatment of osteoarthritis in the first carpometacarpal joint: a double-blind randomized clinical trial. J Orthop Sci. 2014 Sep;19(5):737–43.
18. Topol GA, Reeves KD, Hassanein KM. Efficacy of dextrose prolotherapy in elite male kicking-sport athletes with chronic groin pain. Arch Phys Med Rehabil. 2005;86(4):697–702.
19. Topol GA, Reeves KD. Regenerative injection of elite athletes with career-altering chronic groin pain who fail conservative treatment: a consecutive case series. Am J Phys Med Rehabil. 2008 Nov;87(11):890–902.

20. Eslamian F, Amouzandeh B. Therapeutic effects of prolotherapy with intra-articular dextrose injection in patients with moderate knee osteoarthritis: a single-arm study with 6 months follow up. Ther Adv Musculoskeletal Dis. 2015 Apr;7(2):35–44.
21. Reeves KD, Grasso R, Johnson LL, Rabago D, Topol GA, Podesta LA, et al. Chondrogenic effect of intra-articular hypertonic-dextrose (Prolotherapy) in severe knee osteoarthritis. PM&R. 2016 Nov;8(11):1072–82.
22. Rabago D, van Leuven L, Benes L, Fortney L, Slattengren A, Grettie J, et al. Qualitative assessment of patients receiving Prolotherapy for knee osteoarthritis in a multimethod study. J Altern Complement Med. 2016 Dec 1;22(12):983–9.
23. Rezasoltani Z, Taheri M, Mofrad MK, Mohajerani SA. Periarticular dextrose prolotherapy instead of intra-articular injection for pain and functional improvement in knee osteoarthritis. J Pain Res. 2017;10:1179–87.
24. Hassan F, Trebinjac S, Murrell WD, Maffulli N. The effectiveness of prolotherapy in treating knee osteoarthritis in adults: a systematic review. Br Med Bull. 2017 Jun 1;122(1):91–108.
25. Krstičević M, Jerić M, Došenović S, Jeličić Kadić A, Puljak L. Proliferative injection therapy for osteoarthritis: a systematic review. Int Orthop (SICOT). 2017 Apr;41(4):671–9.
26. Topol GA, Podesta LA, Reeves KD, Raya MF, Fullerton BD, Yeh H. Hyperosmolar dextrose injection for recalcitrant Osgood-Schlatter disease. Pediatrics. 2011 Nov;128(5):e1121–8.
27. Alternative treatments. Dealing with chronic pain. Mayo Clinic health letter (English ed.) 2005 Apr;23(4):1.
28. Hauser RA, Lackner JB, Steilen-Matias D, Harris DK. A systematic review of dextrose Prolotherapy for chronic musculoskeletal pain. Clin Med Insights: Arthritis Musculoskeletal Disord. 2016 Jul 7;2016(9):139–59.
29. Kim B. The effect of Prolotherapy for the chronic pain of musculoskeletal system. J Korean Academy of Rehabilitation Med. 2001 February;25:128–33.
30. Yelland MJ, Sweeting KR, Lyftogt JA, Ng SK, Scuffham PA, Evans KA. Prolotherapy injections and eccentric loading exercises for painful Achilles tendinosis: a randomised trial. Br J Sports Med. 2011 Apr;45(5):421–8.
31. Maxwell NJ, Ryan MB, Taunton JE, Gillies JH, Wong AD. Sonographically guided Intratendinous injection of hyperosmolar dextrose to treat chronic Tendinosis of the Achilles tendon: a pilot study. Am J Roentgenol. 2007 Oct 1;189(4):W215–20.
32. Ryan M, Wong A, Taunton J. Favorable outcomes after Sonographically guided Intratendinous injection of hyperosmolar dextrose for chronic Insertional and Midportion Achilles Tendinosis. Am J Roentgenol. 2010 Apr 1;194(4):1047–53.
33. Lee JH, Kim E. Autologous platelet-rich plasma versus dextrose Prolotherapy for the treatment of chronic recalcitrant plantar fasciitis. PM&R. 2014 Feb;6(2):152–8.

7 Platelet Rich Plasma

This chapter gives an overview of Platelet Rich Plasma and covers the definition of PRP, its history, mechanism of action, and how to assess the platelet function in the context of PRP.

In the mechanism of action, the role of various granules in the secretion of the different growth factors like TGF, PDGF, IGF, FGF, and VEGF are discussed. The importance of fibrin scaffold in the maintenance of the concentration of growth factors also touched upon. The importance of intraosseous injection of PRP in osteoarthritis of the knee, the role of tenocytic stem cells, SNARE protein and the role of Calcium inactivation are also discussed. Finally, insight into the principle involved in the test of assessing the platelet function is also looked upon with mentioning of LTA test.

7.1 Definition

Platelet Rich Plasma (PRP) is defined as the volume of autologous plasma with a platelet concentration well above the baseline. The normal average platelet count in whole blood is around 200,000/μL, so the platelet counts in PRP should average 1,000,000/μL [1, 2].

7.2 History

Around 40 odd years, back platelets were considered as mere clotting factors. All that changed in 1974, when Ross et al. gave new insights into the pathogenesis of atherosclerosis. They found that either the addition of intact platelets and calcium or supernatant derived from activated platelets resulted in the mitogenic activity [3].

The term Platelet-Derived Growth Factors (PGDF) was coined by Witte et al. in 1978 [4]. In subsequent decades various platelet-derived factors namely, Transforming Growth Factor Beta (TGFβ), Insulin-Like Growth Factors (IGF),

S. Trebinjac, M. K. Nair, *Regenerative Injections in Sports Medicine*,
https://doi.org/10.1007/978-981-15-6783-4_7

Basic Fibroblast Growth Factors (bFGF), Vascular Endothelial Growth Factors (VEGF), were identified. The discovery of these factors paved the way for non-hemostatic therapy of platelets. By the late 1990s, the term " Regenerative Medicine" was coined [5].

Regeneration or in situ repair can be achieved if necessary raw material is provided. The three essential components needed for tissue regeneration are cells, growth factors, and scaffold. PRP is included under regenerative medicine as it can provide growth factors and scaffolds necessary for tissue regeneration [6].

The first published clinical report on PRP was in 1998 by oral surgeons incorporating PRP into cancellous bone graft for mandibular defects [7]. Ever since the use of PRP in dental and maxillofacial surgeries increased significantly. Nowadays, PRP is considered as a valuable adjunct in many ablative surgical procedures such as mandibular reconstructions, periodontal surgeries, osteomyelitis, osteoradionecrosis, to name a few [8]. Recently PRP is proposed for the management of bisphosphonate-related osteonecrosis of the jaw (BRONJ) [9]. It is used widely in sports injuries, orthopedics, traumatology, and dentistry [10].

7.3 Mechanism of Action

Platelets are non-nucleated cellular components present in the whole blood along with white and red blood cells. They are cytoplasmic fragments of megakaryocytes which are formed in the bone marrow. The platelets are smaller than other blood cells measuring about 2 μm in diameter. Normal platelet count in a healthy human being ranges from 150,000 to 350,000 per microlitre (μL). Along with fibrin, platelets are important in the hemostatic function of the blood.

Platelets contain a lot of proteins, cytokines, and other biological factors. More than 300 proteins are identified to be released from platelets, the concentration of some are low (Thrombospondin) and some are high (platelet glycoprotein V) [11]. Many growth factors are released by the granules in platelets. There are three main types of granules in platelets; Alpha (α) granules, dense granules, and lysosomes. Among these granules, α and dense granules are present only in platelets and megakaryocytes (Fig. 7.1).

There is an average of 80 α granules in each platelet and they outnumber dense granules [13]. Dense granules contain small molecules like serotonin, ADP, and phosphate, whereas the α granules contain proteins including hemostatic factors such as Factor V, VWF, fibrinogen; angiogenic factors like angiogenin, VEGF; anti-angiogenic factors like angiotensin, PF4; growth factors like PGDF, bFGF, SDF 1α; proteases like MMP2, MMP9; necrotic factors like TNF α, TNF β, and cytokines [14] (Table 7.1).

Platelet growth factors along with plasma growth factors and fibrin stimulate cell proliferation and migration, synthesis and deposition of extracellular matrix components, angiogenesis and tissue remodeling [16] So when PRP is injected, it delivers growth factors into the tissues and at the same time simulates and amplifies the

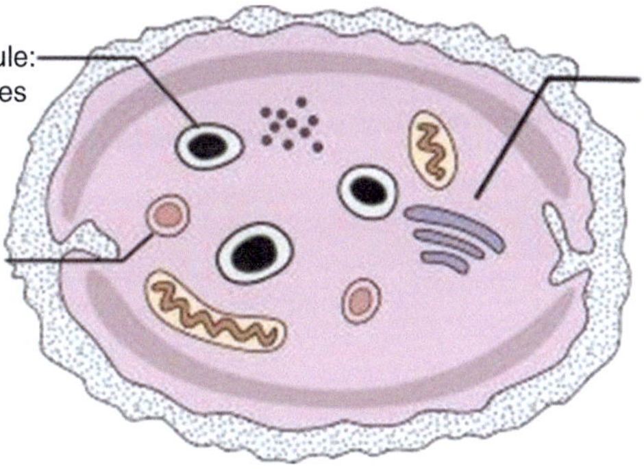

Fig. 7.1 Platelet granules. Figure from [12] with permission Available via license: CC BY 4.0

Table 7.1 Growth factors present in Platelet Rich Plasma (PRP) and their functions [15]

Name of Growth Factors	Functions
Transforming growth factor beta-1; TGFB1	Proliferation, differentiation, in many cell types
Platelet-derived growth factor, alpha polypeptide; PDGFA	Potent mitogen for connective tissue cells
Platelet-derived growth factor, beta polypeptide; PDGFB	Promotes cellular proliferation, inhibits apoptosis
Platelet-derived growth factor C; PDGFC	Increase in the motility of different cells (mesenchymal cells, fibroblasts, smooth muscle cells, capillary endothelial cells, neurons)
Platelet-derived growth factor D; PDGFD	Plays a role in developmental and physiologic processes and in a disease like cancer, fibrotic diseases, and arteriosclerosis
Insulin-like growth factor I; IGF1	Mediates growth-promoting effects of growth hormone
Fibroblast growth factor I; FGF1	Induces liver gene expression, angiogenesis, and fibroblast proliferation
Epidermal growth factor; EGF	Induces differentiation of specific cells, act as a potent mitogenic factor for a variety of cultured cells
Vascular endothelial growth factor A; VEGFA	Primarily a mitogen for vascular endothelial cells induces angiogenesis
Vascular endothelial growth factor B; VEGF B	Regulator of blood vessel physiology, a role in endothelial targeting of lipids to peripheral tissues
Vascular endothelial growth factor C; VEGFC	Angiogenesis and endothelial cell growth, and also affect the permeability of blood vessels

spontaneous healing response in injured areas (Fig. 7.2). The fibrin scaffold is generated in situ and it interacts with extracellular matrix proteins and cells binding with fibronectin. This produces a transient three-dimensional scaffold, which gradually releases and maintains the concentration of growth factors at the scaffold [16] (Fig. 7.3).

There are various application techniques adopted to enhance the efficacy of PRP depending upon the clinical condition. PRP is injected into tissues like muscles,

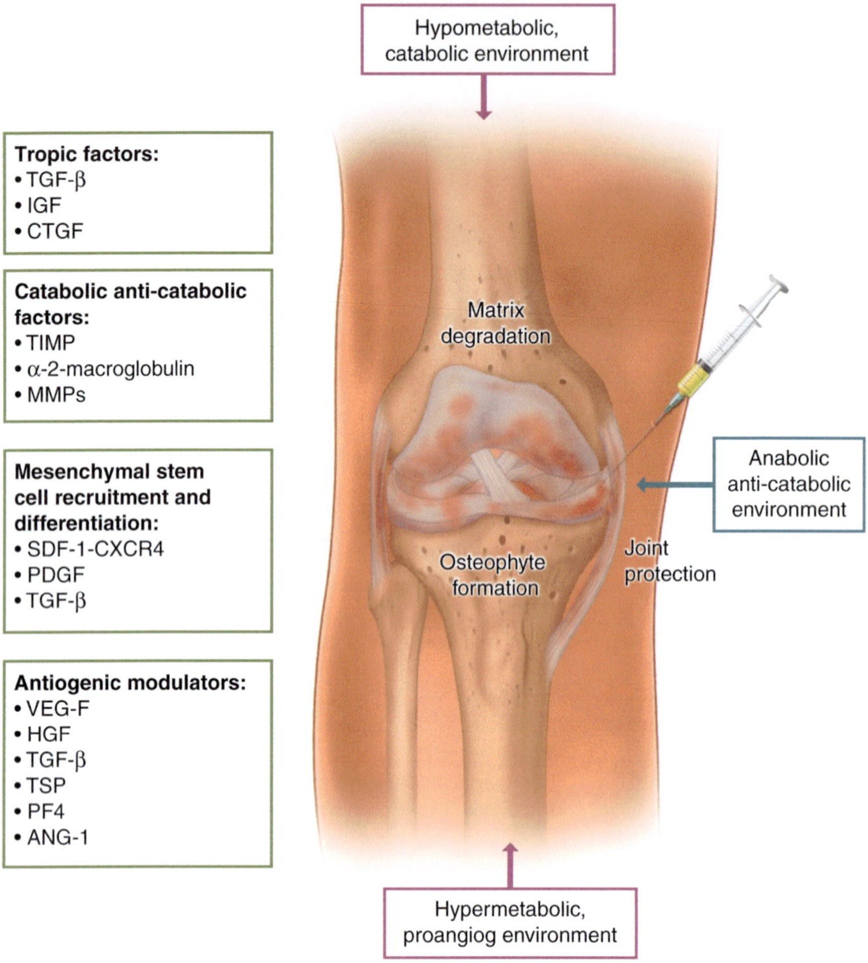

Fig. 7.2 Mechanism of action of PRP in Knee Osteoarthritis with permission from [17]

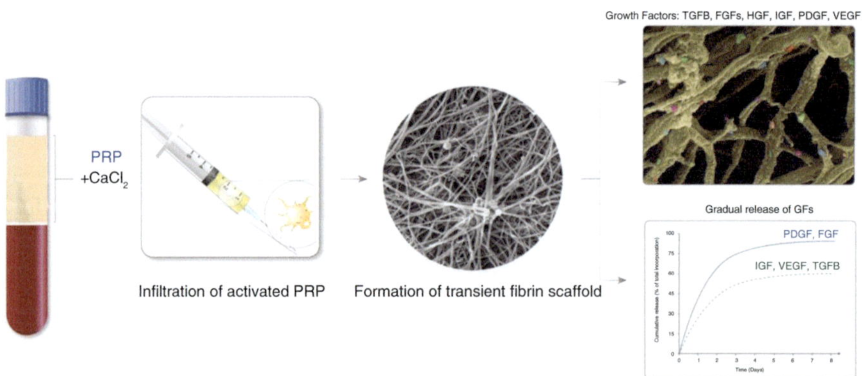

Fig. 7.3 Explaining the release of GF after injecting into the tissues. Fig from [16] with permission

tendons, and ligaments to enhance the healing. It is a common practice to inject PRP in degenerative joint conditions like osteoarthritis of the knee. The initiating factors in osteoarthritis are believed to be a malfunction of the whole joint than in the cartilage alone. So infiltration of PRP in the joint space alone is not sufficient to find a solution to this problem. It has been found that the lesion in the subchondral bone initiates a cross-talk between it and the cartilage resulting in the disruption of the joint homeostasis and inflammation of the joint [16]. Because of this insight, intraosseous infiltration of PRP is proposed as a target for treatment. When PRP is injected intraosseous, growth factors get access to this area and in the deep layers of the cartilage which is otherwise non-accessible in intra-articular infiltration. It stimulates the synthesis of hyaluronic acid and lubricin by synoviocytes and chondrocytes. It also helps in homing and chondrogenic differentiation of mesenchymal stem cells of subchondral bone and synovial fluid. On the other hand, it suppresses the NF-κβ pathway activation [16] (Fig. 7.4).

Proliferation of tenocytes helps in healing injured tendons. But the healing potential of this mechanism is not optimal as the proliferation rate of tenocytes and blood supply to tendons is limited. In in vitro studies, the ability of PRP to promote tenocyte proliferation was demonstrated [18]. In addition to tenocytes, tendons also contain Tendon Specific Stem Cells which constitute about 5% of the tendon cells. The Tendon specific Stem Cells have a high proliferation rate and platelet rich clot release accelerates their proliferation. PRP is found to increase the proliferation of circulating bone marrow and adipose-derived stem cells, which in turn helps in tendon healing [18].

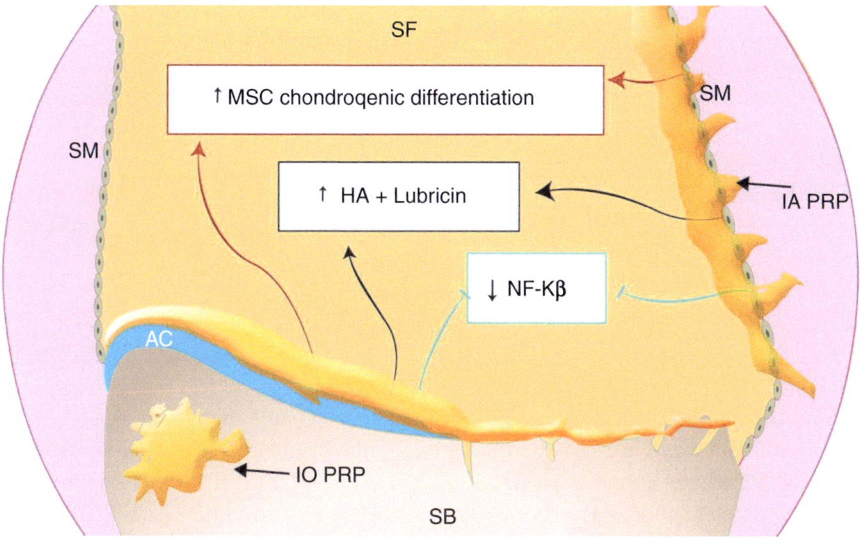

Fig. 7.4 Intraosseous (IO) and intra-articular (IA) infiltration of PRP—mechanism of action: from [16] with permission. *SM* Synovial Membrane, *SB* Subchondral Bone, *AC*, Articular Cartilage, *SF* Synovial Fluid, *HA* Hyaluronic Acid, *MSC* Mesenchymal Stem Cells, *NF-κβ* Nuclear Factor kappa-light-chain-enhancer of activated β cells

Even though platelets have secretory properties, unlike other secretory cells they do not synthesize the materials stored in their granules [19]. The secretion of the contents of these granules occurs through exocytosis and a receptor mechanism (*S*oluble *N*SF (N-ethylmaleimide-sensitive factor) *A*ttachment protein *Re*ceptors—SNARE) [13]. The main SNARE protein responsible is syntaxin 4 for α granule secretion and syntaxin 2 for dense granules. In addition to these, there are second messengers responsible for platelet secretion, such as Ca + and activated protein kinase C (PKC). The platelet cells are activated by specific ligands attached to the membrane receptors. This triggers the cleavage of certain molecules, which in turn result in increased intracellular Ca + concentration, which induces exocytosis [13]. The whole mechanism of platelet secretion is poorly understood until now.

Within 10 min of clotting, the platelets start actively secreting these proteins and within an hour, more than 95% of the pre-synthesized growth factors are secreted [20]. After the initial burst of secretion of growth factors, platelets synthesize and secrete additional factors for several days in their life [20].

Various methods are used to delay the release of growth factors from platelets. One such method is the addition of Calcium Chloride ($CaCl_2$). The addition of $CaCl_2$ results in the formation of a dense fibrin matrix. Intact platelets are trapped in this matrix and release growth factors slowly over a period of 7 days. The fibrin matrix is also found to contribute to healing by acting as a scaffold for cell migration and new matrix formation [15].

In order to have its full potential, platelets rich plasma has to be developed in an anticoagulated state. Once it is developed and kept sterile it would remain viable for nearly 8 h [20]. The anticoagulated serum is re-coagulated by the addition of $CaCl_2$. The intrinsic coagulation pathway is activated by factor 8 and prothrombin is converted to thrombin by Ca+, which in turn converts fibrinogen to fibrin. This leads to cross-linking and clotting. The thrombin is known to activate platelets via specific subtypes of protease-activated receptors [21]. As the clotting process activates the platelets, the growth factors are secreted from the cell through the cell membrane. The granules fuse to the cell membrane and the growth factors are converted into a bioactive state by the addition of histones and carbohydrate side chains. The growth factors thus secreted are attached to the cell membrane of the target sites (graft, flap, or wound) via transmembrane receptors. Platelets that are damaged or become nonviable by the processing will not be able to secrete the bioactive growth factors [20]. It is found out that adult mesenchymal cells, osteoblasts, fibroblasts, endothelial cells, and epidermal cells express the cell membrane receptors to growth factors in PRP [20].

But there are instances where one of these mechanisms might fail. A set of disorders characterized by absent or empty granules in platelets is categorized as Platelet storage pool disorders (SPDs) [22]. One of the disorders is Human α SPD or Gray platelet syndrome where there is a marked reduction of α granules and the tendency for bleeding [23].

7.4 Assessment of Platelet Function

There are many testing systems and equipment available for platelet function ranging from simple testing of bleeding time by Duke method to advanced testing like light transmission aggregometry (LTA). The majority of these testing systems are meant for whole blood, but the LTA is found to be useful exclusively for PRP sample testing for platelet function. LTA was developed in the 1960s by Born and is considered as the gold standard for platelet function [24], In the LTA test, the ability of platelet aggregation in response to external agents (viz adenosine diphosphate (ADP), arachidonic acid (AA), collagen, and epinephrine) are measured in vitro. The test is based on light transmission through the samples of PRP after the addition of an exogenous agonist. The PRP sample becomes clearer after the addition of agonists as it helps in precipitation of the platelets. This allows more light to pass through the sample. The device records the rate of transmission and percentage of increase from 0% to 100% by a photometer. This is converted into a graph with the help of a computer [25]. This method is widely used to detect platelet function disorders and monitor antiplatelet therapies. LTA is the first diagnostic step in evaluation of platelet disorders by various studies [25]. Aggregation of 60% or more is considered as normal [26] (Fig. 7.5). But the assessment of platelet functions is not practiced in Regenerative Injections with PRP, but done more in haematology applications.

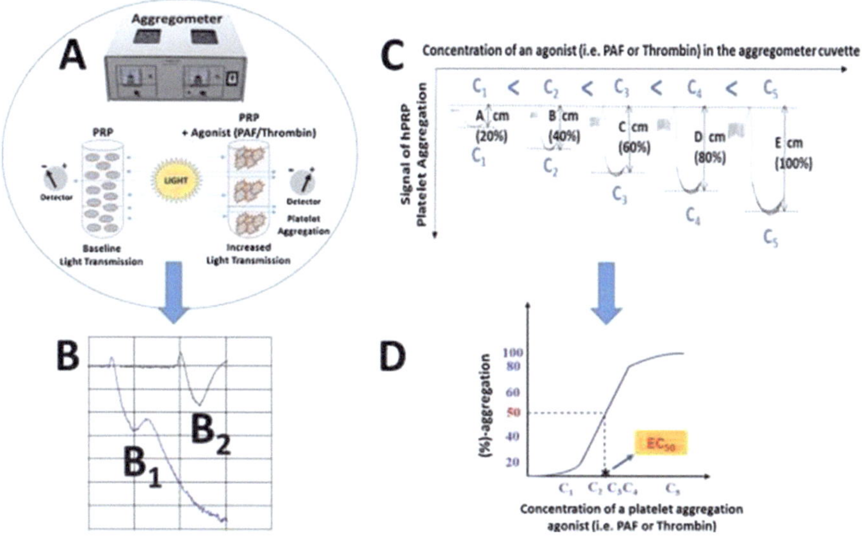

Fig. 7.5 Application of LTA assay to evaluate agonists in platelet aggregation of PRP. Fig from [27] Creative Commons CC-BY license.

The assessment of platelet function using whole blood aggregation by impedance method was developed later and found to be superior to the optical one [26]. But in this technique whole blood is used than with PRP, so it might be useful in the assessment of platelet function for the individual, not necessarily checking the function of platelets in the sample to be injected.

Key Points

- Concentration of platelets in PRP is much higher than that found in plasma.
- PRP can provide growth factors and scaffolds necessary for tissue regeneration.
- When PRP is injected, it delivers growth factors into the tissues and also simulates and amplifies the spontaneous healing response in injured areas.
- Calcium chloride found to delay the release of growth factors from platelets.
- PRP injection to muscles, tendons, and ligaments helps to enhance the healing. PRP found to help in tenocyte proliferation of tendons.
- Intra osseous infiltration of PRP found to be more beneficial than intra-articular injection in Osteoarthritis.
- Platelets have secretory granules that contain growth factors and secretion of these granules are mediated through SNARE proteins but the whole mechanism of their function is not yet fully understood.
- Assessment of platelet function by the LTA method might be useful in determining the quality of PRP injected.

References

1. Alves R, Grimalt R. A review of platelet-rich plasma: history, biology, mechanism of action, and classification. Skin Appendage Disord. 2018 Jan;4(1):18–24.
2. Orsini JA. Equine emergencies. 4th ed. St. Louis, Mo: Elsevier; 2014.
3. Ross R. Atherosclerosis–an inflammatory disease. N Engl J Med. 1999 Jan 14;320(2):115–26.
4. Witte L, Kaplan K, Nossel H, Lages B, Weiss H, Goodman D. Studies of the release from human platelets of the growth factor for cultured human arterial smooth muscle cells. Circ Res. 1978 Mar;42(3):402–9.
5. Haseltine WA. Interview: commercial translation of cell-based therapies and regenerative medicine: learning by experience. Regen Med. 2011 Jul 1;6(4):431–5.
6. Lana JFSD, Andrade Santana MH, Dias Belangero W, Malheiros Luzo AC. Platelet-rich plasma: regenerative medicine: sports medicine, orthopedic, and recovery of musculoskeletal injuries. 2014th ed. Berlin, Heidelberg: Springer; 2013.
7. Marx RE, Carlson ER, Eichstaedt RM, Schimmele SR, Strauss JE, Georgeff KR. Platelet-rich plasma: growth factor enhancement for bone grafts. Oral Surg Oral Med Oral Pathol Oral Radiol Endod. 1998 Jun;85(6):638–46.
8. Shaikh ZS, Thompson AR, Halsnad M, Fowell CJ, Millar BG, Grew NR, Pigadas N. The clinical applications of platelet-rich plasma in oral and maxillofacial surgery. Br J Oral Maxillofac Surg. 2011;49:S98.
9. Albanese A, Licata ME, Polizzi B, Campisi G. Platelet-rich plasma (PRP) in dental and oral surgery: from the wound healing to bone regeneration. Immun Ageing. 2013 Jan 1;10(1):23.
10. Ficek K, Kamiński T, Wach E, Cholewiński J, Cięszczyk P. Application of platelet rich plasma in sports medicine. J Hum Kinet. 2011 Dec 1;30(1):85–97.
11. Coppinger JA, Cagney G, Toomey S, Kislinger T, Belton O, McRedmond JP, et al. Characterization of the proteins released from activated platelets leads to localization of novel platelet proteins in human atherosclerotic lesions. Blood. 2004 Mar 15;103(6):2096–104.

12. de Jong JSG, LRC D. Platelets and cardiac arrhythmia. Front Physiol. 2010;1:166.
13. Reed G. Platelet secretory mechanisms. Semin Thromb Hemost. 2004 Aug;30(4):441–50.
14. Heijnen HF, Debili N, Vainchencker W, Breton-Gorius J, Geuze HJ, Sixma JJ. Multivesicular bodies are an intermediate stage in the formation of platelet alpha-granules. Blood. 1998 Apr 1;91(7):2313.
15. Sánchez-González DJ, Méndez-Bolaina E, Trejo-Bahena NI. Platelet-rich plasma peptides: key for regeneration. Int J Pept. 2012;2012:532519–0.
16. Milano G, Sánchez M, Jo CH, Saccomanno MF, Thampatty BP, Wang JH. Platelet-rich plasma in orthopaedic sports medicine: state of the art. J ISAKOS: Joint Disord Orthop Sports Med. 2019 Jul;4(4):188.
17. O'Connell B, Wragg N, Wilson S. The use of PRP injections in the management of knee osteoarthritis. Cell Tissue Res. 2019 May 6;376(2):143–52.
18. Zhou Y, Wang JH-C. PRP treatment efficacy for Tendinopathy: a review of basic science studies. Biomed Res Int. 2016 Jan 1;2016:9103792–8.
19. Rendu F, Brohard-Bohn B. The platelet release reaction: granules' constituents, secretion and functions. Platelets. 2001;12(5):261–73.
20. Marx RE. Platelet-rich plasma: evidence to support its use. J Oral Maxillofac Surg. 2004;62(4):489–96.
21. Toyoda T, Isobe K, Tsujino T, Koyata Y, Ohyagi F, Watanabe T, et al. Direct activation of platelets by addition of CaCl2 leads coagulation of platelet-rich plasma. Int J Implant Dent. 2018 Dec;4(1):1–11.
22. Rao A, Jalagadugula G, Sun L. Inherited defects in platelet signaling mechanisms. Semin Thromb Hemost. 2004 Oct;30(5):525–35.
23. Raccuglia G. Gray platelet syndrome: a variety of qualitative platelet disorder. Am J Med. 1971;51(6):818–28.
24. Paniccia R, Priora R, Liotta AA, Abbate R. Platelet function tests: a comparative review. Vasc Health Risk Manag. 2015;11:133–48.
25. Choi J-L, Li S, Han J-Y. Platelet function tests: a review of progresses in clinical application. Biomed Res Int. 2014;2014:456569–7.
26. Dyszkiewicz-Korpanty AM, Frenkel EP, Sarode R. Approach to the assessment of platelet function: comparison between optical-based platelet-rich plasma and impedance-based whole blood platelet aggregation methods. Clin Appl Thromb Hemost. 2005 Jan;11(1):25–35.
27. Tsoupras A, Zabetakis I, Lordan R. Platelet aggregometry assay for evaluating the effects of platelet agonists and antiplatelet compounds on platelet function in vitro. MethodsX. 2019;6:63–70.

Platelet Rich Plasma: Preparation Methods

8

This chapter gives an overall idea about PRP preparation techniques, the difference between single and double spin methods, activation techniques, calculation of platelet capturing efficiency using various formulas, different classifications systems and brief about different types of platelet products. The chapter does not go into in-depth analysis of each and every product available in the market and also does not cover surgical applications of PRP.

There are different protocols available for PRP preparation and different types of kits available in the market by various manufacturers, each claiming theirs' superior.

Generally, all protocols involve the collection of blood (Fig. 8.1), centrifuge the sample (either single or double centrifuge) (Figs. 8.2, 8.3, and 8.4), subjecting it to temperature or not, and activating the platelets with exogenous factors or without it. Procedures differ in the volume of blood collected, force and duration of centrifugation, single step or two steps centrifugation, and the resulting volume of platelets. The concentration of platelets also varies depending upon the protocols used (Table 8.1).

The double spin method found to yield a higher concentration of platelets compared to a single spin [3].

According to Yin et al. centrifugation at 160 xg for 10 min or 250 xg for 15 min found to remove the buffy coat and would provide pure PRP [4].

Whatever the methods of preparation of platelets, the following calculations are used to express the characteristics of platelets in Platelets Containing Plasma (PCP) and pure Platelet Rich Plasma (p-PRP) [4].

$$\text{Platelet Capture Efficiency}\left(\%\right)=\frac{\begin{array}{l}\textit{The volume of PCP or p}-\textit{PRP in mL}\\ \times\ \textit{Platelet concentration in PCP or p}-\textit{PRP}\left(10^{9}/L\right)\end{array}}{\begin{array}{l}\textit{Volume of whole blood}\left(mL\right)\\ \times\ \textit{Platelet Concentration of whole blood}\left(10^{9}/L\right)\end{array}}$$

S. Trebinjac, M. K. Nair, *Regenerative Injections in Sports Medicine*,
https://doi.org/10.1007/978-981-15-6783-4_8

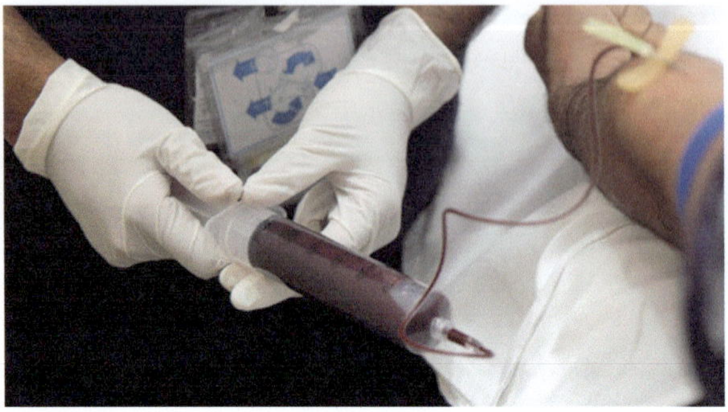

Fig. 8.1 Withdrawal of blood

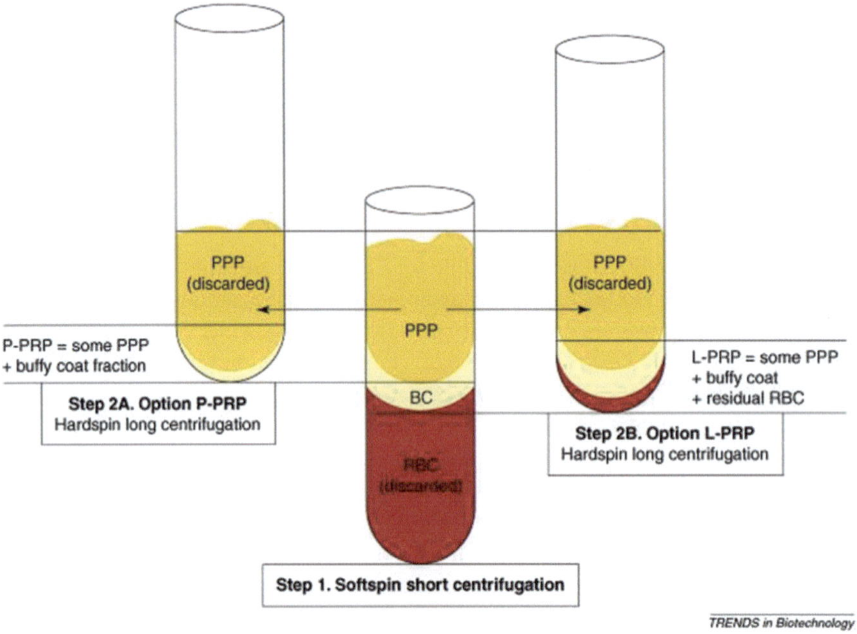

Fig. 8.2 Classical manual Platelet Rich Plasma protocol using two-step centrifugation: from [1] with permission *P-PRP* Pure Platelet Rich Plasma, *L-PRP* Leukocyte, and Platelet Rich Plasma, *PPP* Platelet Poor Plasma, *B.C.* Buffy Coat, *RBC* Red Blood Cells

$$\text{Platelet Enrichment Factor}\left(\text{fold}\right)=\frac{Platelet\ Concentration\ in\ PCP\ or\ p-PRP\left(10^{9}/L\right)}{Platelet\ Concentration\ of\ Whole\ Blood\left(10^{9}/L\right)}$$

$$\text{Leukocyte reducing efficiency}\left(\%\right)=100-\frac{\begin{array}{l}Volume\ of\ PCP\ or\ p-PRP\ in\ mL\\ \times\ Leukocyte\ Concentration\ of\ PCP\ or\\ p-PRP\left(10^{9}/L\right)\end{array}}{\begin{array}{l}The\ volume\ of\ whole\ blood\ in\ mL\\ \times\ Leukocyte\ concentration\ in\\ whole\ blood\left(10^{9}/L\right)\end{array}}$$

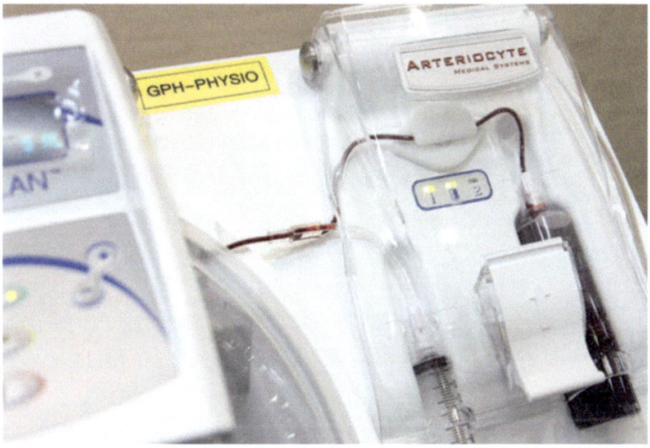

Fig. 8.3 Blood with syringe in centrifuge

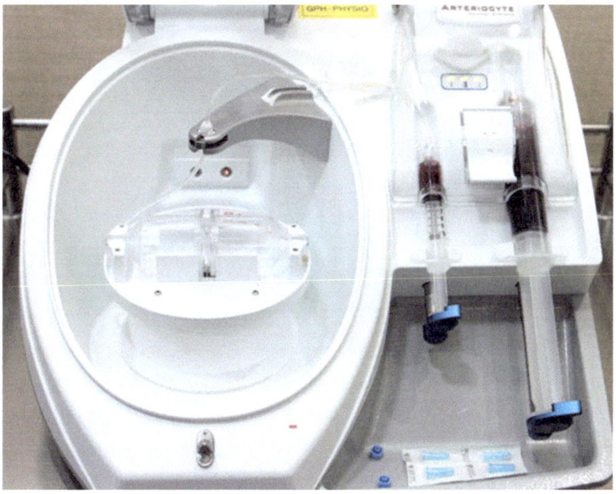

Fig. 8.4 Collection of PRP during centrifuge

$$\text{Erythrocyte Reducing Efficiency}(\%) = 100 - \frac{\begin{array}{l} \textit{Volume of PCP or p} - \textit{PRP in mL} \\ \times \textit{Erythrocyte Concentration of PCP or} \\ \textit{p} - \textit{PRP}\left(10^{12}/L\right) \end{array}}{\begin{array}{l} \textit{Volume of whole blood in mL} \\ \times \textit{Erythrocyte concentration in} \\ \textit{whole blood}\left(10^{12}/L\right) \end{array}}$$

8.1 Activation of Platelets

There are different methods available in practice for the activation of platelets in PRP. PRP activated with $CaCl_2$ found to release significantly higher concentration of growth factors, compared with thrombin or $CaCl_2$/thrombin combination or with

Table 8.1 Summarizing single and double spin methods, from [2] with permission

Single Spin Systems							
Manufacturer	Type of system	Centrifugal force (g)		Centrifuge duration (Min)		Whole blood volume mL	Final volume of PRP in mL
ACP	Plasma	350		5		11	2–5
GPS 3	Buffy coat	1100		15		54	6
Eldoret	Unknown	580		8		9	2
Regen PRP	Leukocyte reduced	1500		5		8	4
Double spin systems							
Manufacturer	Type of system	Centrifuge force (g) first spin	Centrifuge force (g) second spin	Centrifuge duration (min) first spin	Centrifuge duration (min) second spin	Whole blood volume mL	Final volume of PRP in mL
Cascade	Plasma	1100	1450	6	15	9	2
GLO	Buffy coat	1200	600	5	2	9	0.6
Smart prep	Buffy coat	1250	1050	14	7–10	60	Unknown
KYOCERA	Unknown	600	2000	7	5	20	2
Magellan	Buffy coat	610	1240	4	6	60	3
Prosys	Unknown	1660	2008	3	3	30	3

nonactivated PRP. The concentration of growth factors released was different with different activation agents. $CaCl_2$/thrombin combination produced higher growth factor release in the first hour compared with $CaCl_2$ alone or type 3 collagen alone, whereas $CaCl_2$ alone produced the highest growth factor release over a 24 h period [5].

8.2 Classifications of PRP Preparations

There are different classification systems existing in the literature based upon the PRP preparation methods and cellular parameters. The widely used classification systems are the PRP method and the Buffy coat method [3].

The first-ever scientific classification was done in 2008 by Ehrenfest, Rasmusson, and Albrektsson which is considered a milestone in PRP classification [1]. This was a simple classification taking two parameters into account; the presence of cell content and fibrin architecture in the preparation. This classified the PRP into 4 groups:

1. *Pure Platelet Rich Plasma (P-PRP) or Leukocyte Poor Platelet Rich Plasma:* Products without leukocytes and low-density fibrin network after activation. The products under this category can be liquid solutions or activated gel forms.
2. *Leukocyte- and Platelet Rich Plasma (L-PRP):* Preparations with leukocytes and low-density fibrin after activation. Like the P-PRP, the products of this category can be liquid solutions or activated gel forms. Many commercial products are available under this category, such as Regen- PRP, Proteal, Arthrex.
3. *Pure Platelet Rich Fibrin (P-PRF)—or Leukocyte-Poor Platelet Rich Fibrin—* Preparations without leukocytes and with a high-density fibrin network. They exist only in a strongly activated gel form and hence cannot be injected or used like traditional fibrin glues. Fibrinet System (Surgeon-defined Graft (SDG) and Platelet Rich Fibrin Matrix (PRFM) Membrane) are some of the examples.
4. *Leukocyte- and Platelet Rich Fibrin (L-PRF)*: Products with leukocytes and high-density fibrin network. Like P-PRF these also exist only in a strongly activated gel form and hence cannot be injected or used like traditional fibrin glues.

Classifications used for sports medicine

1. Sports Medicine Classification (Mishra Classification): Takes into consideration platelet and leukocyte concentration [6] (Table 8.2).
2. PAW Classification (Delong et al): [7] (Table 8.3) (Fig. 8.5).
3. PLRA Classification (Mautner et al): [8].

Depends on the following parameters (Table 8.4)

- Platelet concentration (absolute number of platelets/μL)
- Leukocyte concentration, including the concentration of neutrophils
- Red blood cell concentration
- Activation by exogenous agents

Table 8.2 Mishra classification

Classification	White blood cells	Activation	Platelet concentration
Type 1	Increased	No activation	A– ≥5x B– <5x
Type 2	Increased	Activated	A– ≥5x B– <5x
Type 3	Minimal or no WBCs	No activation	A– ≥5x B– <5x
Type 4	Minimal or no WBCs	Activated	A– ≥5x B– <5x

Table 8.3 PAW Classification

Platelets	P1(≤baseline)	P2(>baseline–750,000 cells/μl)	P3(>750,000–1,250,000 cells/μl)	P4 (>1,250,000 cells/μl)
Activation	Exogenous-X		Endogenous	
WBCs				
Total	Above baseline-A		Below baseline-B	
Neutrophils	Above baseline-α		Below baseline-β	

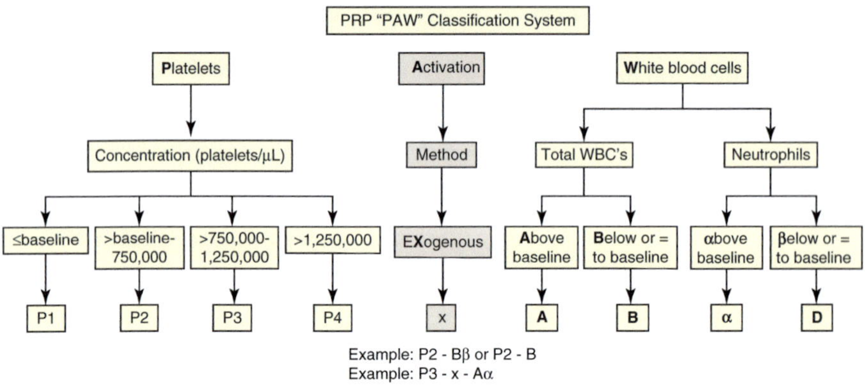

Fig. 8.5 PAW Classification: from [7] with permission

Table 8.4 PLRA classification

Criteria		Final Score	
P	Platelets	P Volume injected	M cells/μL
L	Leukocytes (if white blood cells are present (+), the percentage of neutrophils should also be reported)	>1% <1%	+ –
R	RBCs	>1% <1%	+ –
A	Activation (the method of exogenous activation should be reported)	Yes No	+ –

4. DEPA Classification (Magalon et al): [9].

   This classification is based on the following four parameters (Table. 8.5)

- The dose of injected platelets
- Efficiency of production
- The purity of PRP obtained
- Activation process.

5. MARSPILL (Lana et al): [10].

   This is a more detailed classification mentioning the method of preparation, activation, of platelets done or not, the PRP product is rich or poor in RBCs, spinning is single or double, the number of platelets in the product, PRP is injected under image guidance or not, the concentration of leukocytes in PRP is rich or poor, whether the PRP is light-activated or not (Table 8.6).

Table 8.5 DEPA classification

	Dose of injected platelets (in billions)		Efficiency of process (platelet recovery rate%)		Purity of PRP (relative composition in platelets)	
A	>5	Very high dose	>90	High	>90	Very pure
B	3–5	High dose	70–90	Medium	70–90	Pure
C	1–3	Medium dose	30–70	Low	30–70	Heterogenous
D	<1	Low dose	<30	Poor	<30	Whole blood

Final DEPA score: Expressed as AAA; CAD
For example, the injected platelet is at very high dose and efficiency is high and purity very pure it is expressed as AAA
When platelet is medium-dose efficiency high and purity is very poor (whole blood) it is expressed as CAD

Table 8.6 MARSPILL classification

	Relates to	Type
M	Method	Hand made (H) Machine made (M)
A	Activation	Activated (A+) Not activated (A−)
R	RBCs	Rich (RBC-R) Poor (RBC-P)
S	Spin	One spin (Sp1) Two spin (Sp2)
P	Platelet number (times baseline)	PL 2–3; PL4–6 PL 6–8: PL8–10
I	Image-guided	Guided (G+) Not guided (G−)
L	Leukocyte concentration	Rich (Lc-R) Poor (Lc-P)
L	Light activation	Activated (A+) Not activated (A−)

Reporting as follows: M(H), A(A−), R(RBC-P), S(Sp2), P(PL[4–6]), I(G+), L(Lc-R[2, 3]), L(A−)

8.3 Different Types of Platelet Preparations

8.3.1 Platelet Gel

Platelet Gel (PG) is widely used in orthopedic procedures due to its ease of use compared with recombinant growth factors. It is obtained by adding thrombin and calcium to platelet concentrate to induce the release of growth factors from α granules [11].

The use of Cord Blood Platelet Gel (CBPG) is proposed for regenerative medicine and according to the Italian Health Regulation authority, it is equivalent to adult-derived platelet gel [12].

8.3.2 Comparison of Various PRP and Platelet Lysate

As we have already seen, the method of preparation of PRP is not standardized and many types of kits are available in the market. Some products are high in platelet concentration, some high in leukocyte content, some with higher growth factor concentration.

If the platelet concentration in PRP is less than baseline whole blood values, it may not produce sufficient cellular response, whereas if the concentration is more than sixfold from the baseline, it produces inhibitory effects on healing [13].

Recent investigations by various authors help us to get some insight into these variations.

Magalon et al. compared 5 different PRP preparations in a single-donor model [13]. Comparison was made between Leukocyte rich-PRP from Regen PRP, Mini GPS 3 system, and Leukocyte poor PRP from Selphyl system, Arthrex ACP, and preparation developed in the author's laboratory. The leukocyte rich preparations were having high RBCs, WBCs, and Neutrophils compared with the leukocyte poor PRP.

According to their findings, there were no differences in platelet activation status due to variations in centrifugation time and speeds. There were differences in leukocyte concentrations between leukocyte rich and poor PRP preparations, but the highest leukocyte concentration was only 1.37% in the final PRP preparation.

The higher the volume of blood collected, the higher were the concentration of platelets, growth factors, and platelet and growth factor dosages. The concentration of VEGF and EGF are higher with high WBC count, proving that platelets are not the unique source of growth factors in PRP [14, 15].

The following table shows the different Platelet Rich Products (Table 8.7).

Recent evidence shows that leukocyte rich PRP is beneficial because of its antimicrobial role of PRP treatment [15, 16], whereas high concentration of neutrophils shown to have inhibitory roles in healing due to the release of reactive oxygen species [17].

Table 8.7 Different Platelet Rich Products: adapted from [17] with permission

Type of platelet concentrate	Leukocytes present?	Activation needed?	Status
Leukocyte Platelet Rich Plasma	Yes	Yes/no	Gel/ liquid
Leukocyte Platelet Rich Fibrin	Yes	Yes	Solid
Pure Platelet Rich Plasma	No	Yes/no	Gel/ liquid
Pure Platelet Rich Fibrin	No	Yes	Solid

Key Points

- There are many protocols for the preparation of PRP, but all have collection, centrifugation, and activation.
- Centrifugation is either single spin or double spin.
- Some studies show double spin having higher platelet yield.
- Of the different methods of activation of platelets, $CaCl_2$ found to release a higher concentration of growth factors.
- There are different classifications for PRP preparations and MARSPILL found to be much more comprehensive compared to others.
- Leukocyte rich PRP found to be having antimicrobial effects.
- Platelet Gel and Platelet Rich Fibrin are different types of platelet products used in clinical practice.

References

1. Ehrenfest D, David M, Rasmusson L, Albrektsson T. Classification of platelet concentrates: from pure platelet-rich plasma (P-PRP) to leucocyte- and platelet-rich fibrin (L-PRF). Trends Biotechnol. 2008;27(3):158–67.
2. Oudelaar BW, Peerbooms JC, Rianne HIV, Vochteloo AJH. Concentrations of blood components in commercial platelet-rich plasma separation systems: a review of the literature. Am J Sports Med. 2019 Feb;47(2):479–87.
3. Arshdeep. Platelet-rich plasma by single-spin process in male pattern Androgenetic alopecia: is it an effective treatment? Indian Dermatol Online J. 2017 Nov;8(6):465–7.
4. Yin W, Xu H, Sheng J, Zhu Z, Jin D, Hsu P, et al. Optimization of pure platelet-rich plasma preparation: a comparative study of pure platelet-rich plasma obtained using different centrifugal conditions in a single-donor model. Exp Ther Med. 2017 Sep;14(3):2060–70.
5. Chen X, Jones IA, Park C, Vangsness CT. The efficacy of platelet-rich plasma on tendon and ligament healing: a systematic review and meta-analysis with bias assessment. Am J Sports Med. 2018 Jul;46(8):2020–32.
6. Mishra A, Harmon K, Woodall J, Vieira A. Sports medicine applications of platelet rich plasma. Curr Pharm Biotechnol. 2012 Jun;13(7):1185–95.
7. DeLong JM, Russell RP, Mazzocca AD. Platelet-rich plasma: the PAW classification system. Arthroscopy. 2012;28(7):998–1009.
8. Mautner K, Malanga GA, Smith J, Shiple B, Ibrahim V, Sampson S, Bowen JE. A call for a standard classification system for future biologic research: the rationale for new PRP nomenclature. PM&R. 2015;7(4):S53–9.
9. Magalon J, Chateau AL, Bertrand B, Louis ML, Silvestre A, Giraudo L, et al. DEPA classification: a proposal for standardising PRP use and a retrospective application of available devices. BMJ Open Sport Exerc Med. 2016;2(1):e000060.

10. Lana JFSD, Purita J, Paulus C, Huber SC, Rodrigues BL, Rodrigues AA, et al. Contributions for classification of platelet rich plasma – proposal of a new classification: MARSPILL. Regen Med. 2017;12(5):565–74.
11. Devescovi V, Leonardi E, Ciapetti G, Cenni E. Growth factors in bone repair. Chir Organi Mov. 2008;92(3):161–8.
12. Piccin A, Di Pierro AM, Canzian L, Primerano M, Corvetta D, Negri G, et al. Platelet gel: a new therapeutic tool with great potential. Blood Transfus. 2017 Jul;15(4):333–40.
13. Magalon J, Bausset O, Serratrice N, Giraudo L, Aboudou H, Veran J, Magalon G, Dignat-Georges F, Sabatier F. Characterization and comparison of 5 platelet-rich plasma preparations in a single-donor model. Arthroscopy. 2014;30(5):629–38.
14. Castillo TN, Pouliot MA, Kim HJ, Dragoo JL. Comparison of growth factor and platelet concentration from commercial platelet-rich plasma separation systems. Am J Sports Med. 2011 Feb;39(2):266–71.
15. Moojen DJF, Everts PAM, Schure R, Overdevest EP, van Zundert A, Knape JTA, et al. Antimicrobial activity of platelet-leukocyte gel against Staphylococcus aureus. J Orthop Res. 2008 Mar;26(3):404–10.
16. Bielecki T, Dohan DM, Ehrenfest PA, Everts AW. The role of leukocytes from L-PRP/L-PRF in wound healing and immune defense: new perspectives. Curr Pharm Biotechnol. 2012 Jun;13(7):1153–62.
17. Pavlovic V, Ciric M, Jovanovic V, Stojanovic P. Platelet rich plasma: a short overview of certain bioactive components. Open Med. 2016 Jan 1;11(1):242–7.

9 Clinical Applications of Platelet Rich Plasma in Sports

The aim of this chapter is to present high-quality evidence, available from systematic reviews and meta-analysis related to the efficacy of PRP in sports medicine practice. Considering the high volume of literature, case series and individual RCT studies were avoided. It gives an idea about the role of PRP in muscle, tendon, and ligament injuries. Briefly mentions the higher prevalence of tendinopathy and their mechanism of injury in athletes. Finally, factors influencing the efficacy of PRP injections are also enumerated.

PRP is used in the treatment of soft tissue, joint, and bone issues. It is also a popular treatment among sports professionals and sports physicians as well.

PRP is widely used for ligaments, tendons, muscle issues, which are the most commonly reported problems in sports professionals. In this review, we try to restrict ourselves to sports medicine rather than orthopedic sports surgery applications.

9.1 PRP in Muscle Injuries

Muscle injuries account for about one-third of sports-related injuries. Acute muscle injuries to hamstring are very common among sportspeople, especially professional football and rugby [1, 2]. Hamstring injuries are accounted for about 29% of all sports injuries and up to 50% in sprinters [3].

The conventional approach in management is, ICE (acronym for ice, compression, elevation) RICE (acronym for rest, ice, compression, elevation); PRICE (acronym for protection, rest, ice, compression, elevation) or newly suggested POLICE (acronym for protection, optimal loading, ice, compression, elevation) [4]. The frequent injuries encountered among athletes forces them to be off the training and competition for a longer period of time. This forced the physicians to think about novel treatment approaches hoping to reduce the healing time. PRP is gaining

S. Trebinjac, M. K. Nair, *Regenerative Injections in Sports Medicine*,
https://doi.org/10.1007/978-981-15-6783-4_9

popularity among sports professionals and physicians alike in various sport-related injuries. Despite its popularity, the evidence of its efficacy is conflicting and the jury is still out on this topic.

According to a systematic review published in 2014, promising results were obtained in vivo laboratory studies on animals but there were no convincing results in humans [5]. Similarly, in a systematic review and meta-analysis of RCTs published in 2018, no convincing evidences were found for PRP for muscle injuries [6].

According to the Dutch Hamstring Injection Therapy Study, after 1 year of post-injection, no benefit was observed for intramuscular PRP injections in patients with acute hamstring injury in time for return to play, re-injury rate and changes in subjective, clinical or MRI measures compared to placebo injections [7].

In another systematic review and meta-analysis, Sheth et al. found that PRP improves the time required to return to sport for grade 1 and 2 muscle strain without increasing a re-injury risk in 6 months following. However, when they did a subgroup analysis for hamstring strain the findings were different [8].

In a literature review of Level 1 and 2 studies, Kian et al. found only few Level 1 studies demonstrating a clear benefit, and a large proportion of studies were not blinded or RCT trials [9].

In conclusion, it can be inferred that the benefits of PRP in muscle injuries are not supported by clinical data [10].

9.2 PRP in Tendon and Ligament Pathologies

Tendon and ligament injuries are one of the most prevalent health issues encountered by medical professionals around the world. Annual estimates of patients seeking medical opinion for tendon and ligament injuries in the USA alone are about 16.5 million [11].

Strength per unit area is higher in tendons compared to muscles, but its flexibility is less. So forces generated by muscle may sometimes reach its maximum tendon force and lead to rupture, tear or degeneration. Once it is torn, the tendon has to heal completely to establish its proper fibrillar pattern and alignment of collagen bundles, which usually takes a long time to complete and many times result in inferior quality tendon with scar tissue formation. Even with tendon repair, better outcomes need support from growth factors, mechanical stimulation, tissue engineering, and sometimes, gene therapy [11].

Tendinopathy and tendonitis are common among sportspeople, and they are increasing in prevalence as the number of people participating in sport events increases. Achilles tendinopathy was reported in about 30% of runners, patellar tendinopathy reported about 14% of volleyball players, 13% in handball, 12% in basketball, and 7% in track and field players [12].

Tendinosis occurs due to the imbalance between the demands on the tendon and its capacity for remodeling. Activated platelets release biologically active proteins that promote the recruitment, growth, and morphogenesis of the damaged tissues. Tissue healing is stimulated by enhanced fibroblast migration, proliferation, increased vascularization, and collagen deposition. These are considered as a potential mechanism of tissue healing in tendinosis, which is having a poor intrinsic healing capacity [13].

The fibrillar structure of tendon is made up of Type 1 collagen, whereas type 3 collagen is present in endotenon and epitenon. During the early stages of repair and remodeling, type 3 collagen synthesis is increased and in later phases it is replaced by type 1 collagen (Fig. 9.1). Type 5 collagen is cross-linked to other collagens and it regulates the fibrillar characteristics of the tendon. During the repair process, the collagen is synthesized from tenocytes which are situated in musculotendinous units.

Tenocytes are predominant cells in tendons and they play an important role in tendon repair, but their repair capacity is limited. In addition to tenocytes, tendons also have Tendon Stem Cells (TSC), which are tendon specific adult stem cells, constituting about 5% of cell population [14]. Tendon stem cells are having a high proliferation rate compared with tenocytes.

Laboratory studies have shown that PRP—especially PRP clot release (PRPCR), can promote differentiation of tendon stem cells (TSC) to active tenocytes expressing high proliferation and high collagen production capacities [15].

PRP found to increase collagen synthesis in tenocytes and tendon stem cells and enhance gene expression of type 1 and 3 collagen [14].

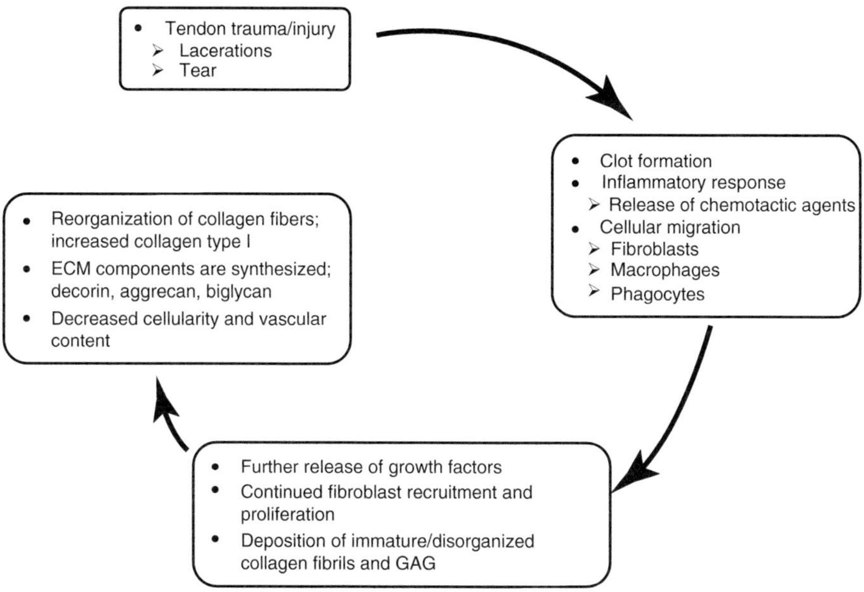

Fig. 9.1 Process of tendon repair: from [11] with permission. *GAG* glycosaminoglycans, *ECM* extracellular matrix

According to the findings of Zang and Wang, PRCR could only induce tendon stem cell differentiation into tenocytes but cannot reverse nontenocyte differentiation, which is prevalent in advanced degenerative tendon pathologies [16]. This could be one of the reasons why PRP does not have much success in treating advanced degenerative tendon pathologies.

In addition to the acceleration of TSC differentiation, PRP accelerates the proliferation of circulating stem cells—bone marrow-derived and adipose derived—and accelerates tendon healing [14]. The concentration of PRP inducing tenocyte proliferation and migration is only up to 1× 10^6 platelets/μL. Above this concentration proliferation and migration found to reduce [17].

In a systematic review and meta-analysis of 37 articles from Level 1 RCT studies, a first of its kind for ligament and tendon injuries, Chen et al. found that PRP showed significant improvement in pain associated with rotator cuff injuries and lateral epicondylitis [18]. The review, from data pooled from 1937 patients, suggests that PRP injections of tendons and ligaments are safe, even though the authors acknowledge there are heterogeneity and possible publication bias as observed by funnel plot.

Miller et al. in a systematic review and meta-analysis showed that there is a level 1 evidence for efficacy of PRP injection in symptomatic tendinopathy [13] (Table 9.1).

According to a systematic review of Level 1-4 studies by Filardo et al., PRP injections were most beneficial in Patellar Tendinopathy. For lateral epicondylitis, PRP was beneficial but could not claim superiority over whole blood injections. Whereas in Achilles tendon pathology, the application of PRP is not indicated either surgically or as a conservative measure. The vast majority of surgical RCTs document a lack of beneficial effect [19].

Table 9.1 Forest plot showing PRP compared with control on tendinopathy pain: from [13] with permission

Study Name	SMD	95% CI		p-Value
Behera, 2015	0.391	0.187	0.594	<0.001
De Jonge, 2011	0.460	0.189	0.730	<0.001
Dragoo, 2014	0.493	0.234	0.752	<0.001
Gautam, 2015	0.426	0.172	0.679	0.001
Gosens, 2011	0.448	0.174	0.722	0.001
Kesikburun, 2013	0.499	0.238	0.760	<0.001
Krogh, 2013a	0.475	0.209	0.740	<0.001
Krogh, 2013b	0.500	0.241	0.759	<0.001
Krogh, 2016	0.504	0.247	0.760	<0.001
Lebiedzinsli, 2015	0.467	0.190	0.745	<0.001
Mishra, 2013	0.469	0.189	0.749	0.001
Montalvan, 2016	0.508	0.250	0.765	<0.001
Palacio, 2016a	0.498	0.239	0.758	<0.001
Palacio, 2016b	0.463	0.198	0.729	<0.001
Rha, 2013	0.450	0.186	0.714	<0.001
Shams, 2016	0.477	0.210	0.754	<0.001
Stenhouse, 2013	0.485	0.221	0.748	<0.001
Yadav, 2015	0.424	0.168	0.680	0.001
TOTAL	0.468	0.215	0.722	<0.001

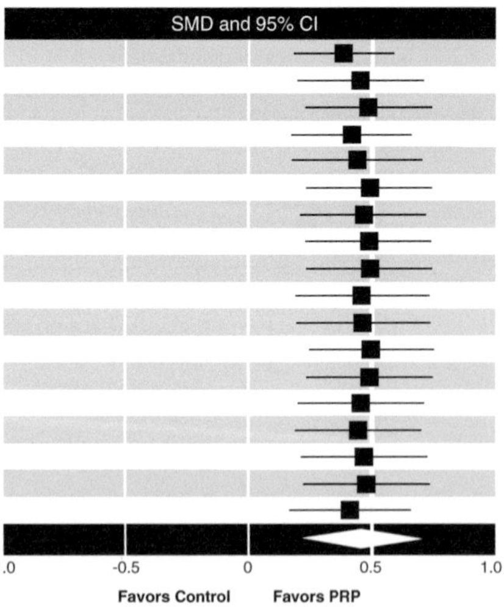

9.3 Anterior Cruciate Ligament Pathology

According to systematic reviews by Taylor et al., addition of PRP is not shown to give any benefit over standard ACL reconstruction procedures [20]. Conversely, another review by Vavken et al. observed the addition of PRP to ACL reconstruction may have a beneficial effect on graft maturation around 20 to 30%. But the quality of this evidence was only Level 3 [21].

In a review article for PRP augmentation in ACL reconstruction, Luca et al. found that intraoperative PRP usage found to be safe as no infections or other complications were observed [22]. PRP found to reduce the surgical morbidity in some studies. Augmentation of PRP in ACL reconstruction patients showed higher neovascularization at least for a period of 4 to 6 weeks and the graft showed more homogenous signal in MRI images at 4 to 12 months post-surgery.

In another systematic review by Di Matteo et al., it was clearly showed that PRP improved graft maturation overtime. The review also observed that 70 to 84% of patients return to previous level of activity without surgery by using PRP in partial ACL tears, but this was based upon two studies [23].

9.4 Rotator Cuff Tendinopathy

Chen et al. did a systematic review and meta-analysis with bias assessment for PRP on tendon and ligament healing. The study followed PRISMA guidelines and included only Level 1 studies. The review included 37 articles and the majority of the articles included were for rotator cuff (38%) and lateral epicondylitis (38%). They found patients treated with PRP had significantly less pain in the long term [18].

In a prospective RCT done by Shams et al. in symptomatic partial rotator cuff tears, comparing subacromial injection of PRP with corticosteroids showed a statistically significant difference between PRP and corticosteroids in pain and functional scales at 12 weeks, favoring PRP treatment, but did not show a difference at 6 months [24].

According to a systematic review by Miranda et al., after analyzing 35 articles (10 laboratory studies, 17 clinical assays, and 8 meta-analyses) concluded there is no solid scientific or clinical evidence supporting the use of PRP in the treatment of Rotator cuff pathology in routine clinical practice [25].

Saltzman et al. did systematic review and meta-analysis to find out whether the use of PRP at the time of surgery improved outcomes in arthroscopic rotator cuff repair. According to their review, use of PRP does not improve clinical outcomes or retear rates [26].

9.5 Patellar Tendinopathy

We have already seen in the above section, systematic review by Filardo et al., PRP injections were found to be most beneficial in Patellar Tendinopathy [19].

Systematic review by Liddle et al. found that PRP is safe and promising therapy in recalcitrant patellar tendinopathy, but could not establish its superiority over physical therapy [27]. Of the 11 studies included in this review, only 2 were RCT, one prospective and the rest were case series.

In another systematic review by Andriolo et al. recommended multiple PRP injections as a suitable option as it offers more satisfactory results at long term follow up. Their recommendations are also based on two RCT studies, 5 prospective case series and two prospective comparative studies [28].

In a meta-analysis of randomized trials Dupley et al. found PRP is better than Extracorporeal Shock Wave Therapy (ESWT) and dry needling at 6 months follow up [29].

9.6 Plantar Fasciitis

In an RCT trial comparing saline with ultrasound-guided PRP injection in 62 adults, Moneim et al. found that it is beneficial in pain and function [30].

In a systematic review and meta-analysis comparing corticosteroids with PRP, Singh et al. found improved pain and function scores in PRP groups at 3 months. A total of ten studies involving 517 patients was involved and assessed with the Cochrane Risk Bias Tool and NewCastle Ottawa Scale (NOS). Pain in Visual Analogue Score (VAS) and American Orthopedic Foot and Ankle Score (AOFAS) were used as outcome scales. Significant differences were observed in VAS and AOFAS at 3 months but no differences noticed at 6 months [31].

9.7 Lateral Epicondylitis

Lateral epicondylitis is one among the tendinopathies in sportspeople, which shows reasonably good results with PRP.

According to the systematic review by Ben Nafa et al., compared with corticosteroid injections, PRP injections demonstrated a long term therapeutic effect, even though short-term rapid effects were observed in the corticosteroid group [32].

Systematic review and meta-analysis done by Arirachakaran et al. to compare corticosteroids, autologous blood (AB) and PRP injections in lateral epicondylitis. According to the findings of this review, there was no statistically significant difference in the visual analog score (VAS) and the Disabilities of Arm Shoulder and Hand (DASH) comparing PRP and AB injections. Higher risk of adverse effects was reported in AB injections than PRP [33].

Darby et al. conducted a systematic review of overlapping meta-analysis comparing different injection treatments for lateral epicondylitis [34]. The objective was to find out which meta-analysis provided the best clinical evidence when comparing injections of corticosteroid, autologous blood and PRP. The study included 9 meta-analyses, of which two were level 1 studies and seven were level 2 studies. There were 8656 patients meeting the eligibility criteria. Quality of the meta-analysis was assessed with the Oxman-Guyatt and Quality of Reporting of Meta-analyses

(QUOROM) systems. The Jadad Decision Algorithm was used to determine the level of evidence for the meta-analysis. Seven meta-analyses found AB and PRP improved pain and function in the 12 to 26 weeks period, whereas 4 studies found corticosteroids reduce pain and improved function in less than 12 weeks period. They also found the highest level of evidence for the Arirachakaran meta-analysis [32] and having the highest quality rating in the Jadad algorithm.

In recalcitrant Lateral epicondylitis, PRP combined with percutaneous needling is found to be an effective treatment for reducing pain, increasing strength and improving function. The study is done in a cohort of 93 patients divided into two groups—fenestration or percutaneous needle tenotomy—and followed up for a period of 3 years [35].

9.8 Ankle Ligaments

Lateral ankle sprain is one of the most common sports injuries encountered in clinical practice. They represent about 85% of the ankle lesions.

The available literature in PRP usage in ankle ligament injuries is sparse. Many are case series and lack level 1 evidence [36, 37].

In an RCT for ultrasound-guided PRP in Antero inferior Tibiofibular Ligament (AITFL) injury in athletes, Laver et al. found benefits in return to play, the reestablishment of syndesmotic joints and less long term residual pain [38].

9.9 Achilles Tendinopathy

Achilles tendon has poor regenerative capacity, and treatment of this condition is difficult. About 30% of runners suffer from Achilles tendinopathy and its annual incidence is between 7-9% [39]. However, according to Fahlstrom, a higher incidence of 40–50% observed in competitive runners [40].

Liu et al., in a meta-analysis of 5 RCTs could not find any difference in Victorian Institute of Sports Assessment-Achilles (VISA-A) between PRP and placebo in chronic Achilles tendinopathy at 12, 24 weeks, and at 1 year. But PRP had better efficacy than placebo at 6 weeks having better VAS scores and tendon thickness at 12 weeks [41].

A meta-analysis by Zhang et al. found no difference between PRP and placebo group in VISA-A score, tendon thickness and color doppler activity in chronic Achilles tendinopathy [42].

9.10 Greater Trochanteric Pain Syndrome (GTPS)

Systematic review of literature by Ali et al. (level1, a systematic review of level1 studies) found PRP injection in GTPS showed significant improvement in 12 months follow-up up and it is a safe and effective treatment [43]. The review was based upon findings of 5 studies, 3 were RCTs, and 2 case series. So high-quality randomized studies with large sample sizes are needed to give further evidence. The HIPPO trial (The Hip Injections PRP versus Placebo) hope to find more answers to this question [44].

9.11 Knee Osteoarthritis

Osteoarthritis of knees is supposed to be higher in sports as higher injury rates predispose the knee to developing OA. As per the systematic review by Driban et al., the overall OA knee prevalence in sports participants was around 7.7% compared with 7.3% in controls. Among the various sports, it is found that soccer players were having the highest prevalence, followed by elite-level long-distance runners, competitive weight lifters, and wrestlers in that order [45]. Erik et al. found that there is a four–sixfold increase in developing knee OA after injury [46]. This systematic review and meta-analysis finding was based upon 53 studies covering about a million population. According to their findings, there is a fourfold increase in developing knee OA after ACL injury and sixfold increase after meniscal injury and combined meniscus and ACL injury when compared with noninjured knee.

PRP found to be effective in symptomatic knee OA, according to the review by Southworth et al. [47].

If we look into systematic reviews and meta-analyses, there are quite a few studies available.

According to the systematic review and meta-analysis from10 trials by Moen et al., intra-articular PRP injections are more effective in reducing pain than placebo, but the level of evidence was limited. But when comparing pain relief with Hyaluronic acid injections, PRP has got moderate evidence. Both these observations were having a high risk of bias. Regarding the function, PRP improved it significantly and the level of evidence was limited to moderate [48]. They updated their review by adding 7 more studies including 1660 participants and found there is moderate evidence to show PRP is more effective than placebo in reducing pain and improving function and superior to Hyaluronic acid [49].

In a meta-analysis of 15 RCTs and 1314 participants, Yanhong Han et al. compared PRP injections with Hyaluronic acid and found PRP reduced pain more effectively than hyaluronic acid and produced better functional improvement at 12 months. Yet they could not recommend the optimal dosage, interval timing, and frequency of injections [50].

In another systematic review and meta-analysis of 18 Level 1 RCTs including 811 participants by Belk et al., found PRP improved clinical outcomes in WOMAC (Western Ontario and McMaster University Osteoarthritis Index) scores, VAS (Visual Analogue Scale) pain score and IKDC (International Knee Documentation Committee) outcomes than Hyaluronic acid. They also found leukocyte poor PRP was associated with significantly better IKDC scores compared with leukocyte rich PRP [51].

There are ongoing clinical trials without the announcement of results so far. One of them is the RESTORE trial. It is a randomized, placebo-controlled trial comparing 3 weekly PRP injections with placebo. The trial is supposed to recruit around 288 participants and the patients will be evaluated for pain and medial tibial cartilage volume in MRIs at 12 months [52].

Shen et al. did a systematic review and meta-analysis including 14 RCTs and 1423 patients found intra articular PRP injections are probably more efficacious than placebo in knee OA. A risk assessment done showed four studies having moderate and ten studies having a high risk of bias. Importantly, PRP injections do not increase the risk of post-injection adverse events [53].

9.12 Variables Affecting the Efficacy of PRP Preparations

As we have seen from the above studies, there are varying outcomes in pain and functional improvement in different clinical conditions. This may be due to factors related to devices used and centrifugation techniques as different methods yield different concentrations and cellular components. In addition to these, Kuffler [54] identified many factors that might contribute to the efficacy of PRP preparations.

The following are some of the contributory factors for the variability of the efficacy of PRP treatment:

- Blood pressure: High blood pressure induces platelets to release factors into the plasma and decreases platelet numbers. So it is recommended to reduce blood pressure before starting PRP treatment.
- Mental and physical stress: Induces platelets to release their factors. Stress also increases blood hormone levels which can interfere with platelet function. Reducing mental and physical stress during treatment would be beneficial in principle for PRP treatment.
- Diet: Diet rich in saturated fats, sugar or simple carbohydrates induces platelet aggregation. Caffeine, quercetin, anthocyanins, and isoflavones can reduce platelet activation.
- Alcohol and smoking: Alcohol consumption causes decreased platelet activation and aggregation and reduced platelet response to thrombin and collagen. Smoking in limited quantities (three cigarettes per day) was found to increase platelet aggregation.
- Pharmaceutical products: Medications like selective serotonin uptake inhibitors (SSRIs), nonsteroidal anti-inflammatory drugs (NSAIDs), antihistamines, antibiotics, tricyclic antidepressants found to suppress normal platelet functions, factor content, and their ability to aggregate. Quinine is found to reduce platelet content.
- Factors Related to PRP Preparation Techniques:
  - Leukocyte Count
  - Glucose content
  - Platelet Activation Methods
- Factors Related to Application of PRP:
  - Injection techniques

- Local anesthetics
- Timing of Injections
- Number of injections.

Key Points

- The Benefits of PRP in muscle injuries are not yet proven.
- PRP clot release (PRPCR) can promote the differentiation of tendon stem cells.
- PRP in tendon and ligament pathologies are safe and effective.
- ACL tendon reconstruction did not provide an additional advantage for PRP but was shown to improve neovascularization, graft maturation and to reduce surgical morbidity.
- In Rotator cuff tears PRP found to be reducing the pain and function. But there is conflicting evidence for its efficacy from a meta-analysis.
- Patellar tendinopathy found to be responding better with PRP but cannot establish superiority over physiotherapy in recalcitrant tendinopathy. Compared with dry needling and shock wave therapy, PRP found to be superior.
- PRP in plantar fasciitis was effective for pain and function at 3 months but does not last up to 6 months.
- Lateral epicondylitis PRP showed long term effects compared with steroids. Compared with autologous blood injections, PRP did not show any difference, except lower adverse effects in PRP.
- In recalcitrant lateral epicondylitis, PRP combined with percutaneous needling found to be an effective treatment.
- Available studies for PRP in ankle injuries are less, but in one systematic review found it is effective in AITFL injury.
- PRP in Achilles tendinopathy found to be not superior to other treatment modalities, its effect on tendon thickness is debatable.
- PRP was found to be effective in greater trochanteric pain syndrome based on one systematic review but needs further proof.
- PRP was found to be more effective than hyaluronic acid injections in reducing pain and improving the function.
- Stress, diet, alcohol, smoking, medications, preparation, and injection techniques are variables contributing to the efficacy of PRP injections.

References

1. Ekstrand J, Healy JC, Waldén M, Lee JC, English B, Hägglund M. Hamstring muscle injuries in professional football: the correlation of MRI findings with return to play. Br J Sports Med. 2012 Feb;46(2):112–7.
2. Brooks JHM, Fuller CW, Kemp SPT, Reddin DB. Incidence, risk, and prevention of hamstring muscle injuries in professional Rugby union. Am J Sports Med. 2006 Aug 1;34(8):1297–306.
3. Ahmad CS, Redler LH, Ciccotti MG, Maffulli N, Longo UG, Bradley J. Evaluation and Management of Hamstring Injuries. Am J Sports Med. 2013 Dec;41(12):2933–47.

4. Bleakley CM. PRICE needs updating, should we call the POLICE? South African J Sports Med. 2016 Jan;22:25(1).
5. Shariff A, Hamid M, Yusof A, Razif Mohamed Ali M. Platelet-rich plasma (PRP) for acute muscle injury: a systematic review. PLoS One. 2014 Jan 1;9(2):e90538.
6. Grassi A, Napoli F, Romandini I, Samuelsson K, Zaffagnini S, Candrian C, et al. Is platelet-rich plasma (PRP) effective in the treatment of acute muscle injuries? A systematic review and meta-analysis. Sports Med. 2018 Apr;48(4):971–89.
7. Reurink G, Goudswaard GJ, Moen MH, Weir A, Verhaar JAN, Bierma-Zeinstra SMA, et al. Rationale, secondary outcome scores and 1-year follow-up of a randomised trial of platelet-rich plasma injections in acute hamstring muscle injury: the Dutch hamstring injection therapy study. Br J Sports Med. 2015;49(18):1206–12.
8. Sheth U, Dwyer T, Smith I, Wasserstein D, Theodoropoulos J, Takhar S, et al. Does platelet-rich plasma lead to earlier return to sport when compared with conservative treatment in acute muscle injuries? A systematic review and meta-analysis. Arthroscopy. 2018;34(1):281–8. e1
9. Setayesh K, Villarreal A, Gottschalk A, Tokish J, Choate W. Treatment of muscle injuries with platelet-rich plasma: a review of the literature. Curr Rev Musculoskelet Med. 2018 Dec;11(4):635–42.
10. Mosca M, Rodeo S. Platelet-rich plasma for muscle injuries: game over or time out? Curr Rev Musculoskelet Med. 2015 Jun;8(2):145–53.
11. James R, Kesturu G, Balian G, Chhabra AB. Tendon: biology, biomechanics, repair, growth factors, and evolving treatment options. J Hand Surg. 2008;33(1):102–12.
12. Ackermann PW, Renström P. Tendinopathy in sport. Sports Health. 2012 May;4(3):193–201.
13. Miller LE, Parrish WR, Roides B, Bhattacharyya S. Efficacy of platelet-rich plasma injections for symptomatic tendinopathy: systematic review and meta-analysis of randomised injection-controlled trials. BMJ Open Sport Exerc Med. 2017 Nov;3(1):e000237.
14. Zhang J. Wang JH-. Platelet-rich plasma Releasate promotes differentiation of tendon stem cells into active Tenocytes. Am J Sports Med. 2010 Dec;38(12):2477–86.
15. Zhou Y, Wang JH-C. PRP treatment efficacy for Tendinopathy: a review of basic science studies. Biomed Res Int. 2016 Jan 1;2016:9103792–8.
16. Zhang J, Wang JH. PRP treatment effects on degenerative tendinopathy - an in vitro model study. Muscles, Ligaments And Tendons Journal. 2014 Jan;4(1):10.
17. Giusti I, D'Ascenzo S, Mancò A, Di Stefano G, Di Francesco M, Rughetti A, et al. Platelet concentration in platelet-rich plasma affects Tenocyte behavior in vitro. Biomed Res Int. 2014;2014:630870.
18. Chen X, Jones IA, Park C, Vangsness CT. The efficacy of platelet-rich plasma on tendon and ligament healing: a systematic review and meta-analysis with bias assessment. Am J Sports Med. 2018 Jul;46(8):2020–32.
19. Filardo G, Di Matteo B, Kon E, Merli G, Marcacci M. Platelet-rich plasma in tendon-related disorders: results and indications. Knee Surg Sports Traumatol Arthrosc. 2018 Jul;26(7):1984–99.
20. Taylor D, Petrera M, Hendry M, Theodoropoulos J. A systematic review of the use of platelet-rich plasma in sports medicine as a new treatment for tendon and ligament injuries. Clin J Sport Med. 2011 Jul;21(4):344–52.
21. Vavken P, Sadoghi P, Murray MM. The effect of platelet concentrates on graft maturation and graft-bone interface healing in ACL reconstruction in human patients: a systematic review of controlled trials. Arthroscopy. 2011 Nov;27(11):1573–83.
22. Andriolo L, Di Matteo B, Kon E, Filardo G, Venieri G, Marcacci M. PRP augmentation for ACL reconstruction. Biomed Res Int. 2015 Jan 1;2015:371746–15.
23. Di Matteo B, Loibl M, Andriolo L, Filardo G, Zellner J, Koch M, et al. Biologic agents for anterior cruciate ligament healing: a systematic review. World J Orthop. 2016 Sep 18;7(9):592–603.
24. Shams A, El-Sayed M, Gamal O, Ewes W. Subacromial injection of autologous platelet-rich plasma versus corticosteroid for the treatment of symptomatic partial rotator cuff tears. Eur J Orthop Surg Traumatol. 2016 Dec;26(8):837–42.

25. Miranda I, Sánchez-Alepuz E, Lucas FJ, Carratalá V, González-Jofre CA. Use of platelet-rich plasma in the treatment of rotator cuff pathology. What has been scientifically proven? Rev Esp Cir Ortop Traumatol. 2017 Jul;61(4):249–58.
26. Saltzman BM, Jain A, Campbell KA, Mascarenhas R, Romeo AA, Verma NN, Cole BJ. Does the use of platelet-rich plasma at the time of surgery improve clinical outcomes in arthroscopic rotator cuff repair when compared with control cohorts? A systematic review of meta-analyses. Arthroscopy. 2015;32(5):906–18.
27. Liddle AD, Carlos R-ME. Platelet-rich plasma in the treatment of patellar Tendinopathy: a systematic review. Am J Sports Med. 2015 Oct;43(10):2583–90.
28. Andriolo L, Altamura SA, Reale D, Candrian C, Zaffagnini S, Filardo G. Nonsurgical treatments of patellar Tendinopathy: multiple injections of platelet-rich plasma are a suitable option: a systematic review and meta-analysis. Am J Sports Med. 2019 Mar;47(4):1001–18.
29. Dupley L, Charalambous CP. Platelet-rich plasma injections as a treatment for refractory patellar Tendinosis: a meta-analysis of randomised trials. Knee Surg Related Res. 2017 Sep 1;29(3):165–71.
30. Moneim Deghady AA, Abdel Hamid MM, Hussein Helal AM, El-Sherif SM, Latief A, Al Sayed H. Platelet-rich plasma in treatment of plantar fasciitis: randomized double-blinded placebo controlled study. J Appl Clin Pathol. 2019;2(1):1.
31. Singh P, Madanipour S, Bhamra JS, Gill I. A systematic review and meta-analysis of platelet-rich plasma versus corticosteroid injections for plantar fasciopathy. Int Orthop. 2017 Jun;41(6):1169–81.
32. Ben-Nafa W, Munro W. The effect of corticosteroid versus platelet-rich plasma injection therapies for the management of lateral epicondylitis: a systematic review. SICOT-J. 2018;4:11.
33. Arirachakaran A, Sukthuayat A, Sisayanarane T, Laoratanavoraphong S, Kanchanatawan W, Kongtharvonskul J. Platelet-rich plasma versus autologous blood versus steroid injection in lateral epicondylitis: systematic review and network meta-analysis. J Orthop Traumatol. 2016 Jun;17(2):101–12.
34. Houck DA, Kraeutler MJ, Thornton LB, McCarty EC, Bravman JT. Treatment of lateral Epicondylitis with autologous blood, platelet-rich plasma, or corticosteroid injections: a systematic review of overlapping meta-analyses. Orthop J Sports Med. 2019 Mar;7(3):2325967119831052.
35. Gaspar MP, Motto MA, Lewis S, Jacoby SM, Culp RW, Lee Osterman A, et al. Platelet-rich plasma injection with percutaneous needling for recalcitrant lateral Epicondylitis: comparison of Tenotomy and fenestration techniques. Orthop J Sports Med. 2017 Dec 1;5(12):2325967117742077.
36. Samra D, Hiller C, Sman A, Rae K, Linklater J, Refshauge K. Effectiveness of a single platelet rich plasma (PRP) injection to promote recovery in rugby players with ankle syndesmosis injury. J Sci Med Sport. 2016;19:e50.
37. Lai MWW, Sit RWS. Healing of complete tear of the anterior Talofibular ligament and early ankle stabilization after autologous platelet rich plasma: a case report and literature review. The Archives of Bone & Joint Surgery. 2018 Mar 1;6(2):146–9.
38. Laver L, Carmont M, McConkey M, Palmanovich E, Yaacobi E, Mann G, et al. Plasma rich in growth factors (PRGF) as a treatment for high ankle sprain in elite athletes: a randomized control trial. Knee Surg Sports Traumatol Arthrosc. 2015 Nov;23(11):3383–92.
39. Wiklander JLJ. Injuries in runners. Am J Sports Med. 1987 Mar 1;15(2):168–71.
40. Fahlström M, Jonsson P, Lorentzon R, Alfredson H. Chronic Achilles tendon pain treated with eccentric calf-muscle training. Knee Surg Sports Traumatol Arthrosc. 2003 Sep;11(5):327–33.
41. Liu C, Yu K, Bai J, Tian D, Liu G. Platelet-rich plasma injection for the treatment of chronic Achilles tendinopathy: a meta-analysis. Medicine. 2019 Apr;98(16):e15278.
42. Zhang Y, Xu S, Gu P, Du J, Cai Y, Zhang C, et al. Is platelet-rich plasma injection effective for chronic Achilles Tendinopathy? A meta-analysis. Clin Orthop Relat Res. 2018 Aug;476(8):1633–41.

43. Ali M, Oderuth E, Atchia I, Malviya A. The use of platelet-rich plasma in the treatment of greater trochanteric pain syndrome: a systematic literature review. J Hip Preservation Surg. 2018 Aug;5(3):209–19.
44. Oderuth E, Ali M, Atchia I, Malviya A. A double blind randomised control trial investigating the efficacy of platelet rich plasma versus placebo for the treatment of greater trochanteric pain syndrome (the HIPPO trial): a protocol for a randomised clinical trial. Trials. 2018 Sep 21;19(1):517.
45. Driban JB, Hootman JM, Sitler MR, Harris K, Cattano NM. Is participation in certain sports associated with knee osteoarthritis? A systematic review. J Athl Train. 2017 Jun 1;52(6):497–506.
46. Poulsen E, Goncalves GH, Bricca A, Roos EM, Thorlund JB, Juhl CB. Knee osteoarthritis risk is increased 4-6 fold after knee injury – a systematic review and meta-analysis. Br J Sports Med. 2019;53:bjsports-100022.
47. Southworth TM, Naveen NB, Tauro TM, Leong NL, Cole BJ. The use of platelet-rich plasma in symptomatic knee osteoarthritis. J Knee Surg. 2019 Jan;32(1):37.
48. Laudy ABM, Bakker EWP, Rekers M, Moen MH. Efficacy of platelet-rich plasma injections in osteoarthritis of the knee: a systematic review and meta-analysis. Br J Sports Med. 2015 May;49(10):657–72.
49. Moen M, Weir A, Bakker E, Rekers M, Laudy G. Efficacy of platelet-rich plasma injections in osteoarthritis of the knee: an updated systematic review and meta-analysis. Osteoarthr Cartil. 2016;24:S520–1.
50. Han Y, Huang H, Pan J, Lin J, Zeng L, Liang G, et al. Meta-analysis comparing platelet-rich plasma vs hyaluronic acid injection in patients with knee osteoarthritis. Pain Med. 2019 Mar 7;20(7):1418–29.
51. Belk JW, Kraeutler MJ, Houck DA, Goodrich JA, Dragoo JL, McCarty EC. Platelet-rich plasma versus hyaluronic acid for knee osteoarthritis: a systematic review and meta-analysis of randomized controlled trials. Am J Sports Med. 2020 Apr 17:36354652090939–363546520909397.
52. Paterson KL, Hunter DJ, Metcalf BR, Eyles J, Duong V, Kazsa J, et al. Efficacy of intra-articular injections of platelet-rich plasma as a symptom- and disease-modifying treatment for knee osteoarthritis - the RESTORE trial protocol. BMC Musculoskelet Disord. 2018 Jul 28;19(1):272.
53. Shen L, Yuan T, Chen S, Xie X, Zhang C. The temporal effect of platelet-rich plasma on pain and physical function in the treatment of knee osteoarthritis: systematic review and meta-analysis of randomized controlled trials. J Orthop Surg Res. 2017;12:–16.
54. Kuffler DP. Variables affecting the potential efficacy of PRP in providing chronic pain relief. J Pain Res. 2018 Dec 1;12:109–16.

Settings for PRP Injections 10

This chapter gives a stepwise account of preparing PRP for injections. It also mentions the setting and equipment needed and differences between open and closed systems.

10.1 Equipment

The preparation of PRP is through two main techniques [1].

Open Technique and Closed Technique (Semi-Closed and Closed).

Open Technique

The main disadvantage of this technique is exposure of the plasma with the environment of the working area which includes pipettes and collection tubes. It is very difficult to assure that the resulting PRP is not contaminated with microorganisms. The main advantage is that this processing method is cheap.

Closed Technique

It involves the use of commercial equipment like blood collection tube kits and centrifuges. The main advantage is the PRP is not exposed to the environment. The cost of equipment is the main disadvantage.

Majority of the medical devices used in a closed system belongs to one of the following types:

1. Blood is drawn into a collection tube that has an anticoagulant and can be used directly to any centrifuge after collection.
2. Medical devices in which blood is collected into a tube which contains an anticoagulant. The centrifugation can be done in any type of centrifuge.
3. Medical devices in which blood is collected into a syringe which is previously filled with an anticoagulant. The blood is transferred into another device that is compatible with the centrifuge supplied by the manufacturer.

S. Trebinjac, M. K. Nair, *Regenerative Injections in Sports Medicine*,
https://doi.org/10.1007/978-981-15-6783-4_10

Table 10.1 Open and closed PRP system. Adapted from [2] with permission

Platelet concentration class	System Open/ Semi-Closed/ Closed	Device name
L-PRP	Closed	Haemonetics MCS+ 9000 cell separator: 995
	Closed	Magellan autologous platelet separator system
	Closed	MyCells
	Closed	RegenPRP
	Semi-Closed	Dr. Shin's system THROMBO KIT
	Semi-Closed	GenesisCS component concentrating system
	Semi-Closed	GLO PRP
	Semi-Closed	GPS III platelet concentrate system
	Semi-Closed	KYOCERA medical PRP kit
	Semi-Closed	Prosys PRS(PRP) bio kit
	Semi-Closed	SmartPReP system
	Open	JP200
	Open	Plateltex
P-PRP	Closed	COBE spectra LRS turbo (with a leukoreduction set)
	Closed	Vivostat PRF
	Semi-Closed	Arthrex ACP
	Semi-Closed	SELPHYL
	Open	PRGF-Endoret

L-PRP Leukocyte platelet rich plasma, *P-PRP* Pure platelet rich plasma.

The PRP preparation depends upon the equipment used and manufacturers' instructions have to be followed.

The following are some of the examples of Open and Closed Systems used for PRP (Table 10.1).

The following pictures demonstrate the steps in collection and processing of PRP.

The important equipments are PRP kits and centrifuge, usually supplied along with the kits by the manufacturing company.

10.2 PRP Centrifuge

There are different types of centrifuges available in the market, and as mentioned before one step and two-steps centrifugation process. Here we show one step centrifugation and closed system (Fig. 10.1).

10.3 PRP Kit (Fig. 10.2)

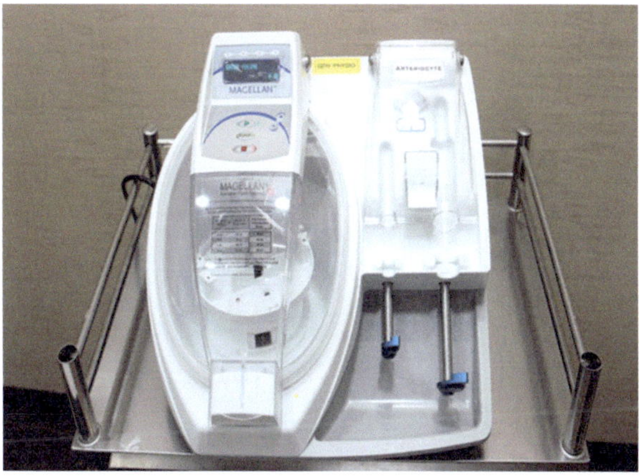

Fig. 10.1 PRP Centrifuge

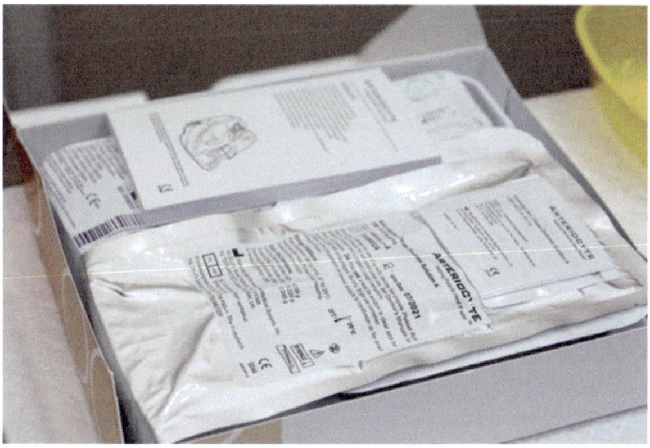

Fig. 10.2 PRP Kit

10.4 Miscellaneous

In addition to kit and the centrifuge, the following are needed for preparation (Figs. 10.3 and 10.4).

- Sterile gown
- Sterile gloves
- Sterile ultrasound gel
- Local anesthetics
- Skin marking pen
- Syringes and needles
- Ultrasound scanner

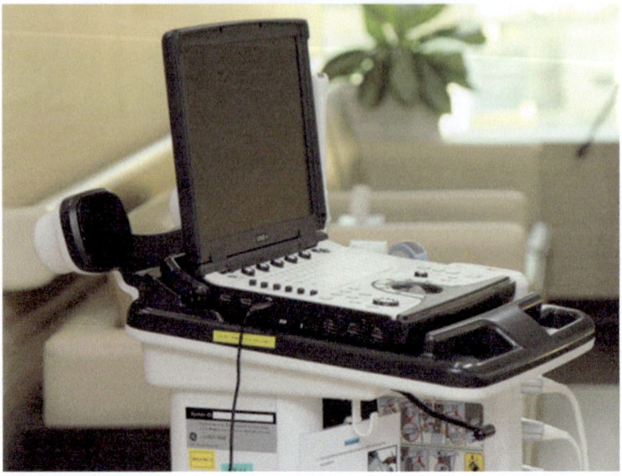

Fig. 10.3 Ultrasound Scanner

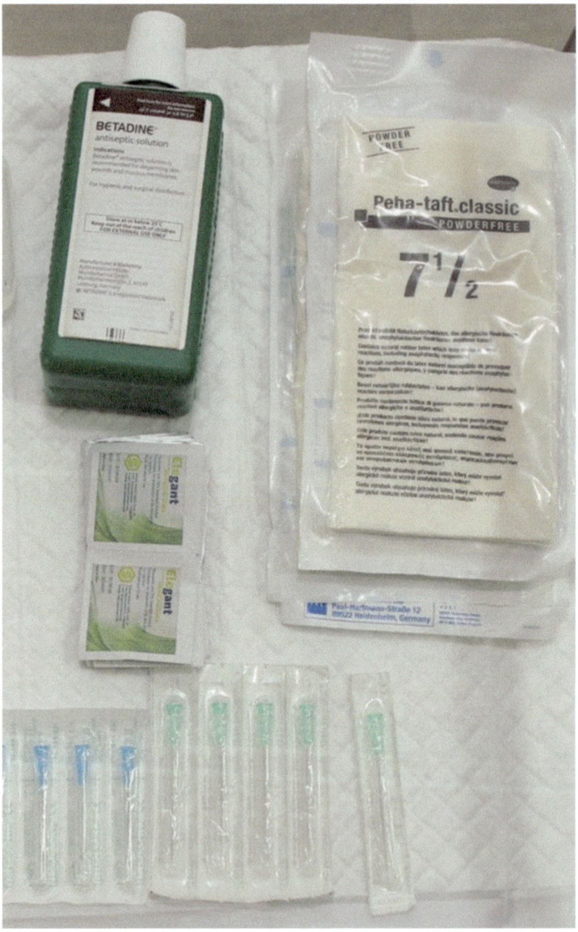

Fig. 10.4 Cleaning solution, gloves, needles

10.5 Steps in Collection

The patient is positioned in a chair or bed and the whole procedure is explained. It makes the patient comfortable and cooperative. The area (usually antecubital vein) is cleaned with isopropyl alcohol and tourniquet is applied. Open the kit and insert the butterfly cannula and once blood starts showing up in the tube, connect the vacutainer or syringe (depending upon the kit). Once the required amount of blood is withdrawn, release the tourniquet and seal the punctured area with adhesive plaster. Transfer the tube to the centrifuge machine or connect the syringe to the machine and spin it for the recommended time. This varies according to the kits and centrifuge. The countrabalance in the machine must be assured (Figs. 10.5, 10.6, 10.7, 10.8 and 10.9).

Once the centrifugation is over, the PRP is ready for injection.

Key Points

- Open and closed systems for PRP preparation are available.
- The closed system is considered superior as there is less chance of contamination.
- Injection should be practiced under aseptic precautions and preferably under image guidance.

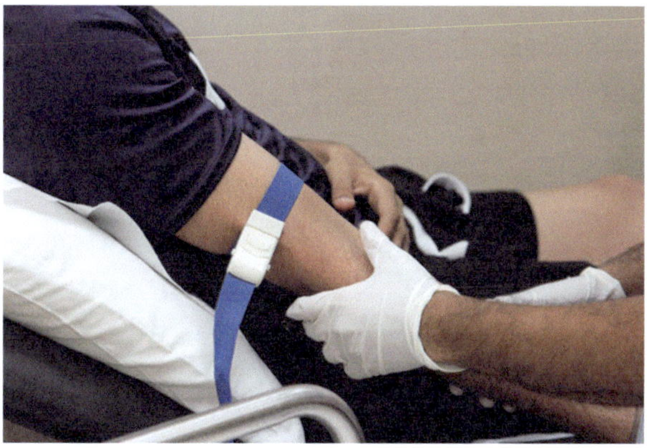

Fig. 10.5 Before Venipuncture: Applying tourniquet and cleaning of the area of antecubital vein for blood collection

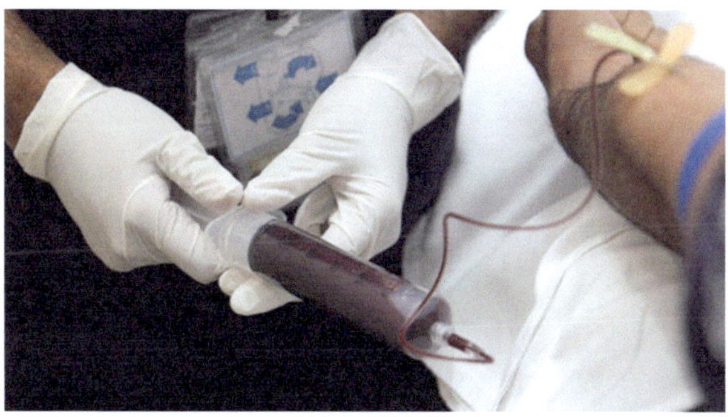

Fig. 10.6 Blood is drawn into syringe

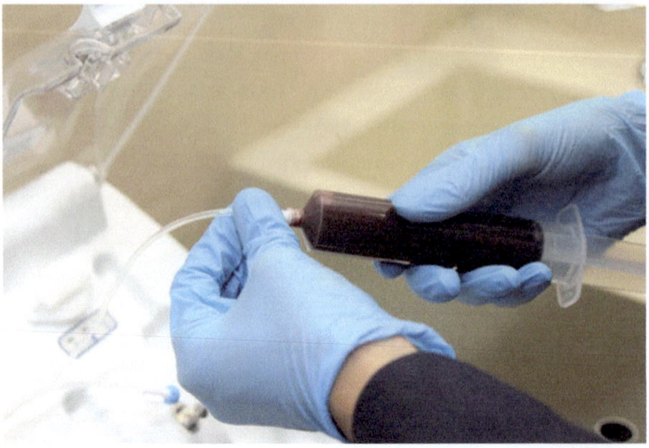

Fig. 10.7 Syringe connected to the centrifuge

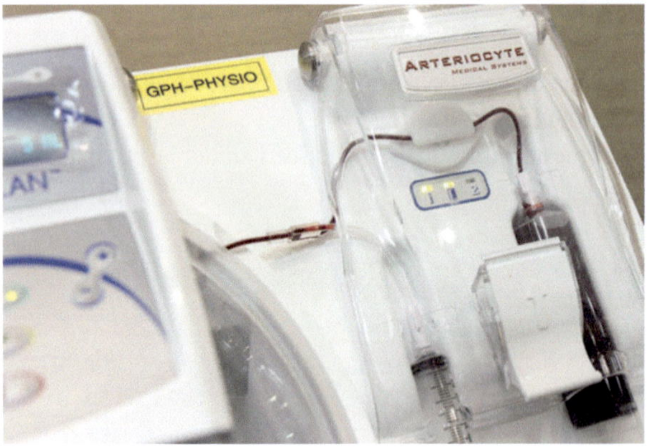

Fig. 10.8 Centrifugation and PRP collection into the empty syringe

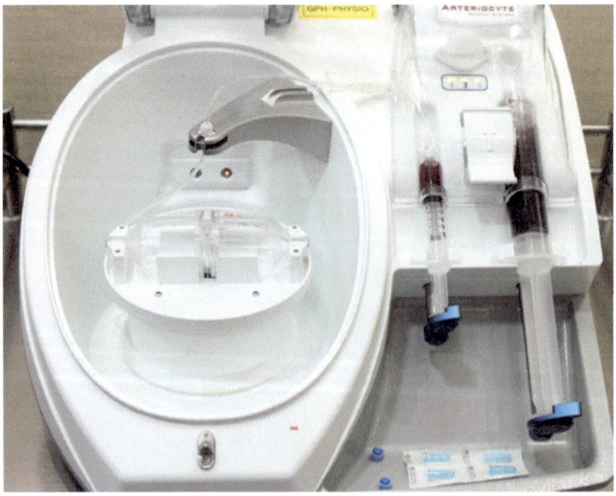

Fig. 10.9 PRP is collected into injection syringe

References

1. Alves R, Grimalt R. A review of platelet-rich plasma: history, biology, mechanism of action, and classification. Skin Appendage Disord. 2018 Jan;4(1):18–24.
2. Pavlovic V, Ciric M, Jovanovic V, Stojanovic P. Platelet rich plasma: a short overview of certain bioactive components. Open Med. 2016 Jan 1;11(1):242–7.

Stem Cells 11

Definition and a brief history of the development of stem cells are described mentioning the names of prominent scientists and their discoveries. It was explained why stem cells attract the attention of scientists and how they can change the paradigm in the management of chronic musculoskeletal injuries. Different types and sources of stem cells, their main features, and potential are pointed out in detail. Limitation and potential hazard in the application of embryonic stem cells are clarified. The benefits of this treatment in the sports field and advantages to other therapies are highlighted. The mechanism of action and complexity of interaction between cells and their environment is discussed. Different theories related to the functioning of cells are described.

11.1 Definition

Stem cells are undifferentiated cells that can divide and differentiate into other types of cells. That means, more specialized cells like cardiac, bone, blood, etc. can be generated from stem cells. Division (self-renewal) and differentiation (specialization into other cells) bring the hope that they might replace damaged tissues in human bodies and restore the function which is partially or completely lost. This assumption brought stem cells into the field of regenerative medicine that has become one of the most attractive medical disciplines in the last 30 years.

11.2 History of Stem Cells

The history of stem cells is long and full of fascination and controversies. There are many scientists who contributed significantly to the development of regenerative medicine. However, we will focus on several important discoveries that marked the modern history of regenerative medicine.

S. Trebinjac, M. K. Nair, *Regenerative Injections in Sports Medicine*,
https://doi.org/10.1007/978-981-15-6783-4_11

One of the most important revelations was the identification of Hematopoietic stem cells in mice (HSC) by Ernest McCulloch and James Till [1]. This discovery paved the way for the treatment of different hematological disorders.

In 1981 the Nobel prize winners Martin Evans and Matt Kauffman were able to isolate, identify, and culture embryonic stem cells (ES) from mouse blastocyst [2].

James Thomson and collaborators did the same from humans [3]. Since the use of embryonic stem cells is considered illegal because the harvesting of it requires destruction or at least manipulation of embryo and it carries the risk of tumor development, immunologic reaction and serious heart problem [4], scientists focused on exploration of adult stem cells of mesenchymal origin.

In 1970 Friedenstein et al. in their original work confirmed that bone marrow possesses the cells that can be differentiated into connective tissues [5]. In current clinical practice, bone marrow becomes one of the main sources of adult stem cells. Minimal criteria for the definition of mesenchymal stem cells in the adult population were first proposed by Potten and Loffler in 1990 [6].

Most of the current research and clinical application is related to adult cells originating from our own body (autologous cells), as they are considered more safe than cells from other sources. However, adult stem cells have lesser differentiation potential and can be used for the regeneration of cells, mainly of mesodermal origin.

In 2006, Japanese scientists Takahashi and Yamanaka, (by inducing four ES cells genes, called "reprogramming factors") were able to reprogram the adult stem cells to create induced pluripotent stem cells (iPSc) [7]. They have similar features to embryonal cells. They used a retrovirus to transfer four important transcription factors (Yamanaka factors) Oct 4, SOX2, cMyc, and Klf4 into the mouse fibroblast cells. IPSc supposed to provide a broader spectrum of potential treatment benefits but they also face similar issues as an ES cells, like teratogenic effects, immunologic reactions, and potential genome instability [4, 8].

11.3 The Main Features of Stem Cells

Stem cells originate from different sources and have different differentiation potential. Depending on their ability to differentiate they might be totipotent, unipotent, oligopotent, pluripotent, and multipotent.

Totipotent cells originate from fertilized eggs, and can differentiate in all types of cells out of embryo. They are used mainly for research purposes but not in clinical practice [9]. Unipotent cells have the lowest differentiation potential and can differentiate along with one germ layer, producing only one type of cell. The skin is an example of unipotent cells. Oligopotent cells can differentiate into a few types of cells. Examples are lymphoid or myeloid cells. Neither unipotent nor oligopotent cells are used in clinical practice. Pluripotent cells originating from the inner cell mass of an embryo (blastocyst) can differentiate into all three germ layers; endoderm, ectoderm, and mesoderm generate different types of cells originating from these layers [10]. Only totipotent cells have larger differentiation potential.

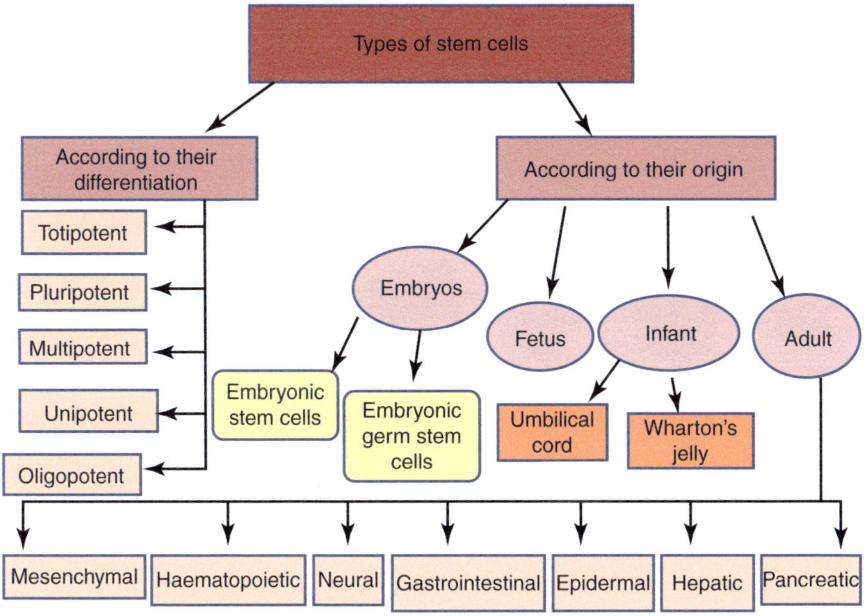

Fig. 11.1 Different type of cells and their sources, from [12] with permission Creative Commons License

Multipotent stem cells can differentiate into more than one type of cell but less than pluripotent cells. They are differentiated mainly into mesodermal layers. The human adult cells, as well as umbilical cord cells, belong to this category. It is possible that there are more sources of multipotent mesenchymal stem cells [11]. Different type of cells and their sources are presented in Fig. 11.1.

The proper recognition of stem cells among the other types of cells is very important to understand their function and possible location. The International Society of Cellular Therapy defined the minimum criteria for recognition of mesenchymal stem cells:

- Adhesion to plastic surface
- Positive expression of protein surface markers CD 73, CD 90, CD 105 (> than 93% expression)
- The absence of hematopoietic markers CD 34, CD 45, CD 14 or CD 11b, CD 79α or CD 19 (< than 2%)
- The absence of HLA Class II molecules
- Differentiation potential into chondrogenic, osteogenic, and adipogenic phenotypes [13]

Division and differentiation are the main features of stem cells. They are able to divide many times and renew themselves for long periods (Fig. 11.2).

This made them unique because already formed cells don't have such an ability. The division of a single cell can produce identical daughter cells. Expansion of the number

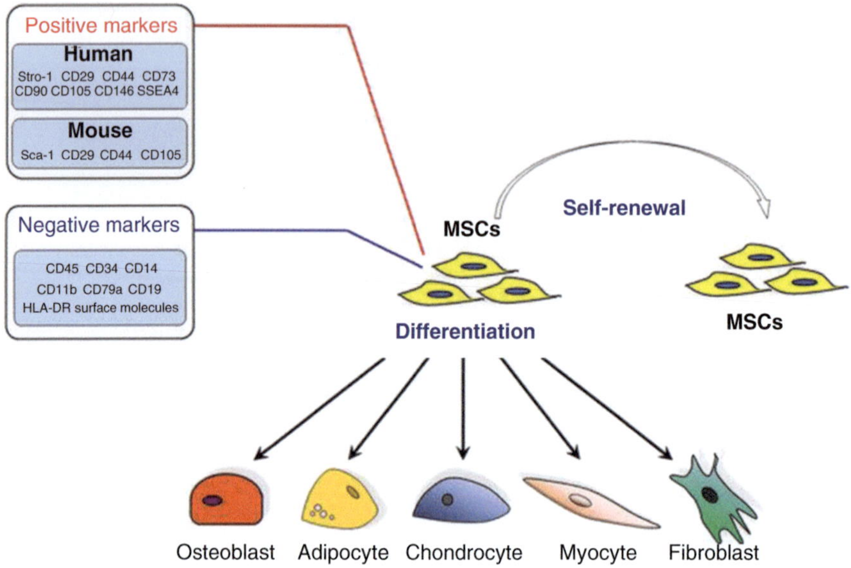

Fig. 11.2 Identification of stem cells by positive and negative markers. The process of self-renewal and differentiation from [14] Creative Commons Attribution License

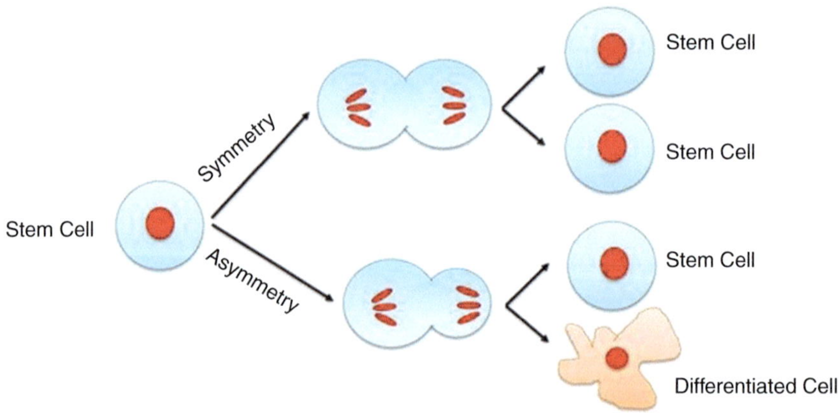

Fig. 11.3 symmetric and asymmetric cell divisionof Stem Cell: from [16] with permission Available via license: CC BY-NC 4.0

of cells by continuing division (a process called proliferation) will produce millions of cells. The division can be symmetric and asymmetric. The symmetric division produces identical cells while asymmetric division will generate nonidentical cells. The balance between symmetric and asymmetric division is very important for repair after injury or disease [15]. Example of symetric and assymetric division is presented in Fig. 11.3.

The process of differentiation is one of the most intriguing events prompting numerous research trials. The microenvironment that promotes stem cell maintenance, so-called "niche" is a particular subject of investigation [17, 18]. It is obvious that a cell's function depends on interaction with other cells located nearby. There is significant progress in a better understanding of common features, structure, and function of stem cells niche, but still insufficient to explain in detail the very complex mechanism of interaction. The future success of stem cell therapy will probably be in proportion to understanding these processes.

11.4 Sources of Stem Cells

Based on origin, stem cells can be classified as embryonic, fetal, adult, and induced pluripotent [19]. Embryonic stem cells (ES) have been derived from the inner cell mass of embryos in the blastocyst stage [20]. They are pluripotent cells able to differentiate into cells originating from all three germ layers; ectoderm, endoderm, and mesoderm. This feature allowed them to produce multiple types of cells [3, 21]. They also have teratogenic effects confirmed in animal studies [3]. Extraction of cells request the destruction of embryos, raising ethical and legal issues. At present, the use of embryonic stem cells for human treatment is considered illegal in most countries. Human fetal stem cells are extracted from amniotic fluid or umbilical cord. They face the same ethical issues as embryonic cells if they are extracted directly from the fetus.

Adult stem cells are multipotent. They can differentiate into the limited type of cells usually in one lineage, e.g., mesoderm. Recent results showed that trans differentiation in other lineages is also possible [22].

There are two types of adult stem cells; hematopoietic stem cells (HSC) that give rise to all types of blood cells (erythrocytes, leukocytes, etc.) and mesenchymal stem cells (MSC) that differentiate into mesodermal structures like cartilage, bone, tendon, ligaments, and adipose tissue [23].

Induced pluripotent cells or reprogrammed adult cells are the subjects of intensive research due to similarity to embryonal cells with possible less risks of adverse reactions [7].

In sports medicine, adult mesenchymal stem cells are the most important because the majority of injuries are related to tissues of mesodermal origin.

MSCs can be extracted from different tissues but most of the time it is from the bone marrow and adipose tissue. However, other sources like the umbilical cord, placenta, etc. can also be used. Self-renewal and proliferation involve a multiple-step process ending up in the maturation of cells and the production of tissues of mesenchymal origin (Fig. 11.4).

The cells extracted from one's own body are called autologous cells, from the other humans (same species) allogenic and different species (animals) xenogenic.

One of the unresolved issues related to the application of mesenchymal stem cells is the lack of consensus about the most valuable source of stem cells for the treatment of cartilage, muscles, ligaments, and tendons. Although cells from different sources share many characteristics specific for MSCs (plastic adherence, specific surface markers expression, ability to differentiate), there are certain differences related to gene expression and cytokine production.

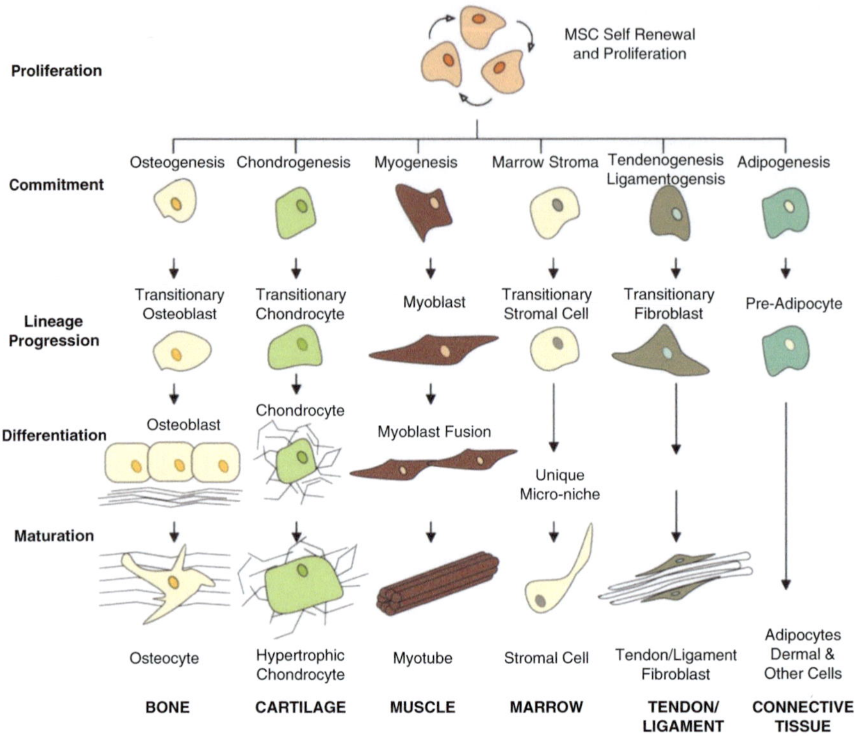

Fig. 11.4 Mesenchymal stem cells proliferation into different lineage. Image from [24] with permission

Comparative analyses of MSCs from bone marrow, adipose tissue, and umbilical cord blood showed that there is no difference in morphology and immunophenotype. But there is a difference in the success rate of isolation of MSCs which is maximal in Bone Marrow (BM) and Adipose Tissue (AT) but not in Umbilical Cord Blood(UCB). However, UCB-MSCs can be cultured longer and have the highest proliferation capacity [25–27]. The raising issue is whether perinatal sources (umbilical cord, placenta, amniotic fluid) produce any viable stem cells after processing [28]. Also, there is a question about the proliferative capacity and osteogenic potential of stem cells in elderly population [29, 30]. It is known that the number and viability of stem cells harvested from the bone marrow declines with age while it stays the same in adipose tissue. It is estimated that adipose tissue possesses 1000 times more MSCs per gram compared to bone marrow [31]. However, according to some in vitro studies, the chondrogenic potential of bone marrow aspirate is higher than from the adipose tissue [32–34].

It is known that the bone marrow or adipose tissue, as well as perinatal sources, are rich in other types of cells that have possible therapeutic effects, so it is difficult to delineate particular effects of stem cells in isolation from others. The potential advantages and disadvantages of different sources of stem cells are listed on Table 11.1.

Table 11.1 Advantages and disadvantages of autologous and allogeneic sources of stem cells

The source of stem cells	Advantages	Disadvantages
Bone marrow	Higher osteogenic and chondrogenic capacity than ADSC.	Invasive donation procedure. Declining numbers due to aging. The lowest proliferation capacity.
Adipose tissue	Higher adipogenic potential than BMAC. Provide much more MSC than bone marrow.	Invasive procedure but more comfortable than bone marrow aspiration.
Umbilical cord	Less invasive procedure, higher proliferation capacity than BM and AT.	Success rate of isolating MSC is lower than BM and AT. Not able to differentiate in adipose tissue. The processing can destroy stem cells.
Amniotic fluid/ membrane	Non-aggressive procedure. Abundant growth factors and other nutrients. The slower release of active factors than PRP, potential longer therapeutic effect.	Majority of stem cells are destroyed during preparation.

11.5 Mechanism of Action

Aside to exhibiting differentiation potential, stem cells are capable to release broad spectrum of trophic substances (cytokines) involved in angiogenesis, anti-inflammatory reactions, immunomodulation and prevention of apoptosis [35].

The exact mechanism of action of stem cells is the subject of intensive research. Initially, it was hypothesized that stem cells after administration can migrate to the injured area, engraft themselves, and start the differentiation process. As a result, the regeneration of damaged tissue is promoted. This hypothesis faced a lot of challenges in experimental work because it doesn't take into account the complexity of the signaling system and specificity of the niche where the cells are embedded [36]. Scientists are trying to get a better insight into the interaction of injected stem cells and their local environment.

Today, most theories estimate the paracrine effects of stem cells with secretion of growth factors, cytokines, and hormones. They play immunomodulatory roles through stimulatory and inhibitory effects. They can inhibit proliferation and activity of natural killer cells, suppress T and B lymphocyte proliferation and dendritic maturation. At the same time, they may induce regulatory T cells. MSCs release soluble factors such as interleukins 6 and 10, prostaglandin E2, hepatocyte growth factor, indoleamine 2,3-dioxygenase, nitric oxide, transforming growth factor β1, human leukocyte antigen, and extracellular vesicles. These factors play a role in immunomodulation [32]. The other possible explanation includes transfer of mitochondria, exosomes or vesicles containing RNA and other different molecules [37], (Fig. 11.5).

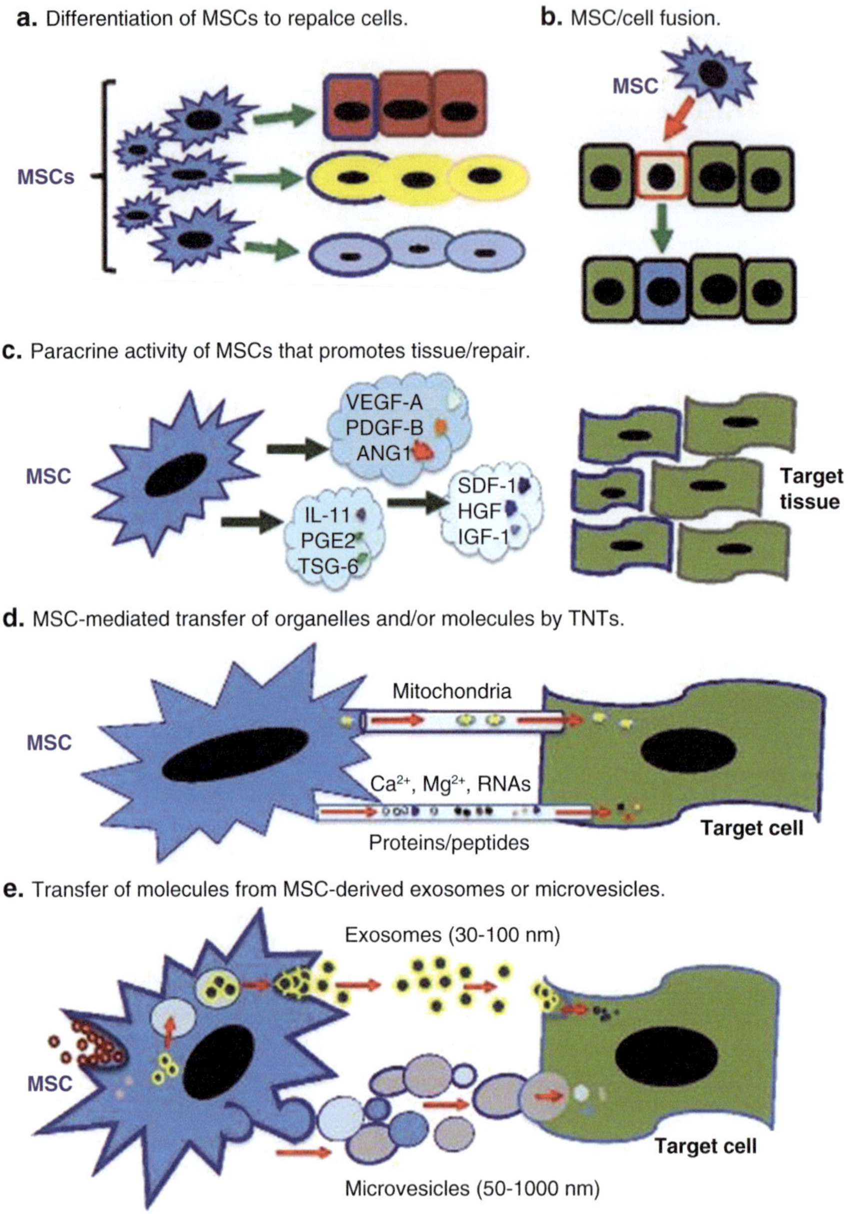

Fig. 11.5 Possible mechanisms of action of MSCs from [37] permission by Creative Commons Attribution 4.0 International License *(*http://creativecommons.org/licenses/by/4.0/*)*

Key Points

- Stem cell discovery changed the paradigm in the management of sports injuries. Their potential to divide and differentiate in other types of cells made them very attractive for scientists, clinicians, and patients.
- The history of stem cells is fascinating and some scientists won the Nobel Prize for their research.
- Unique properties and some positive and negative CD markers are crucial for their recognition among the other cells.
- There are different types of stem cells, extracted from different sources with different regenerative potentials.
- While several theories try to explain possible mechanisms of action of stem cells, the paracrine theory with the secretion of growth factors, cytokines, and hormones is broadly accepted among scientists.

References

1. Becker AJ, McCulloch EA, Till JE. Pillars article: cytological demonstration of the clonal nature of spleen colonies derived from transplanted mouse marrow cells. Nature. 1963. 197:452–454. J Immunol. 2014 Jun 1;192(11):4945–7.
2. Evans MJ, Kaufman MH. Establishment in culture of pluripotential cells from mouse embryos. Nature. 1981 Jul 9;292(5819):154–6.
3. Thomson JA, Itskovitz-Eldor J, Shapiro SS, Waknitz MA, Swiergiel JJ, Marshall VS, et al. Embryonic stem cell lines derived from human blastocysts. Science. 1998 Nov 6;282(5391):1145–7.
4. Yoshihara M, Hayashizaki Y, Murakawa Y. Genomic instability of iPSCs: challenges towards their clinical applications. Stem Cell Rev. 2017 Feb;13(1):7–16.
5. Friedenstein AJ, Chailakhjan RK, Lalykina KS. The development of fibroblast colonies in monolayer cultures of Guinea-pig bone marrow and spleen cells. Cell Tissue Kinet. 1970 Oct;3(4):393.
6. Potten CS, Loeffler M. Stem cells: attributes, cycles, spirals, pitfalls and uncertainties. Lessons for and from the crypt. Development. 1990 Dec 1;110(4):1001–20.
7. Takahashi K, Yamanaka S. Induction of pluripotent stem cells from mouse embryonic and adult fibroblast cultures by defined factors. Cell. 2006;126(4):663–76.
8. Tapia N, Schöler H. Molecular obstacles to clinical translation of iPSCs. Cell Stem Cell. 2016 Sep 1;19(3):298–309.
9. Baker CL, Pera MF. Capturing totipotent stem cells. Cell Stem Cell. 2018 Jan 4;22(1):25–34.
10. Wobus AM, Boheler KR. Embryonic stem cells: prospects for developmental biology and cell therapy. Physiol Rev. 2005 Apr 1;85(2):635–78.
11. Ding D, Shyu W, Lin S. Mesenchymal stem cells. Cell Transplant. 2011 Feb;20(1):5–14.
12. EL Barky AR, Ali EMM, Mohamed TM. Stem cells, classifications and their clinical applications. Am J Pharmacol Ther. 2017;1(1):001–7.
13. Dominici M, Le Blanc K, Mueller I, Slaper-Cortenbach I, Marini FC, Krause DS, et al. Minimal criteria for defining multipotent mesenchymal stromal cells. The International Society for Cellular Therapy position statement. Cytotherapy. 2006;8(4):315–7.

14. Hu L, Yin C, Zhao F, Ali A, Ma J, Qian A. Mesenchymal stem cells: cell fate decision to osteoblast or adipocyte and application in osteoporosis treatment. Int J Mol Sci. 2018 Jan 25;19(2):360.
15. Betschinger J, Knoblich JA. Dare to be different: asymmetric cell division in drosophila, C. elegans and vertebrates. Curr Biol. 2004 Aug 24;14(16):R674–85.
16. Chen X, Ye S, Ying Q. Stem cell maintenance by manipulating signaling pathways: past, current and future. BMB Rep. 2015 Dec;48(12):668–76.
17. Schofield R. The relationship between the spleen colony-forming cell and the haemopoietic stem cell. Blood Cells. 1978;4(1–2):7.
18. Li L, Xie T. Stem cell niche: structure and function. Annu Rev Cell Dev Biol. 2005 Nov 10;21(1):605–31.
19. Brown JC, Shang H, Li Y, Yang N, Patel N, Katz AJ. Isolation of adipose-derived stromal vascular fraction cells using a novel point-of-care device: cell characterization and review of the literature. Tissue Eng Part C Methods. 2017 Mar 1;23(3):125–35.
20. Odorico JS, Kaufman DS, Thomson JA. Multilineage differentiation from human embryonic stem cell lines. Stem Cells. 2001 May;19(3):193–204.
21. Pera MF, Reubinoff B, Trounson A. Human embryonic stem cells. J Cell Sci. 2000 Jan 1;113(1):5.
22. Keilhoff G, Goihl A, Langnäse K, Fansa H, Wolf G. Transdifferentiation of mesenchymal stem cells into Schwann cell-like myelinating cells. Eur J Cell Biol. 2006;85(1):11–24.
23. Caplan AI. Mesenchymal stem cells. J Orthop Res. 1991;9(5):641–50.
24. Firth AL, Yao W, Yuan JXJ. Identification of adult stem and progenitor cells in the pulmonary vasculature. In: Yuan JJ, Garcia J, West J, Hales C, Rich S, Archer S, editors. Textbook of pulmonary vascular disease. Boston, MA: Springer; 2011.
25. Klingemann H, Matzilevich D, Marchand J. Mesenchymal stem cells – sources and clinical applications. Transfus Med Hemother. 2008 Aug;35(4):272–7.
26. Wagner W, Wein F, Seckinger A, Frankhauser M, Wirkner U, Krause U, et al. Comparative characteristics of mesenchymal stem cells from human bone marrow, adipose tissue, and umbilical cord blood. Exp Hematol. 2005;33(11):1402–16.
27. Friedman R, Betancur M, Boissel L, Tuncer H, Cetrulo C, Klingemann H. Umbilical cord Mesenchymal stem cells: adjuvants for human cell transplantation. Biol Blood Marrow Transplant. 2007;13(12):1477–86.
28. Wexler SA, Donaldson C, Denning-Kendall P, Rice C, Bradley B, Hows JM. Adult bone marrow is a rich source of human mesenchymal 'stem' cells but umbilical cord and mobilized adult blood are not. Br J Haematol. 2003 Apr;121(2):368–74.
29. D'Ippolito G, Schiller PC, Ricordi C, Roos BA, Howard GA. Age-related Osteogenic potential of Mesenchymal stromal stem cells from human vertebral bone marrow. J Bone Miner Res. 1999 Jul;14(7):1115–22.
30. Oreffo R, Bennett A, Carr A, Triffitt J. Patients with primary osteoarthritis show no change with ageing in the number of Osteogenic precursors. Scand J Rheumatol. 1998;27:415–24.
31. Aust L, Devlin B, Foster SJ, Halvorsen YDC, Hicok K, du Laney T, et al. Yield of human adipose-derived adult stem cells from liposuction aspirates. Cytotherapy. 2004 Jan;6(1):7–14.
32. Kohli N, Wright KT, Sammons RL, Jeys L, Snow M, Johnson WEB. An in vitro comparison of the incorporation, growth, and Chondrogenic potential of human bone marrow versus adipose tissue Mesenchymal stem cells in clinically relevant cell scaffolds used for cartilage repair. Cartilage. 2015 Oct;6(4):252–63.
33. Afizah H, Yang Z, Hui JHP, Ouyang H, Lee E. A comparison between the Chondrogenic potential of human bone marrow stem cells (BMSCs) and adipose-derived stem cells (ADSCs) taken from the same donors. Tissue Eng. 2007 Apr;13(4):659–66.
34. Mohamed-Ahmed S, Fristad I, Lie SA, Suliman S, Mustafa K, Vindenes H, et al. Adipose-derived and bone marrow mesenchymal stem cells: a donor-matched comparison. Stem Cell Res Ther. 2018 Jun 19;9(1):168.

35. Konala VBR, Mamidi MK, Bhonde R, Das AK, Pochampally R, Pal R. The current landscape of the mesenchymal stromal cell secretome: a new paradigm for cell-free regeneration. Cytotherapy. 2015;18(1):13–24.
36. Iso Y, Spees JL, Serrano C, Bakondi B, Pochampally R, Song Y, et al. Multipotent human stromal cells improve cardiac function after myocardial infarction in mice without long-term engraftment. Biochem Biophys Res Commun. 2007;354(3):700–6.
37. Spees JL, Lee RH, Gregory CA. Mechanisms of mesenchymal stem/stromal cell function. Stem Cell Res Ther. 2016 Aug 31;7(1):125.

Stem Cells: Preparation Methods 12

The technique of harvesting and processing of mesenchymal stem cells from two main sources, bone marrow, and adipose tissue are explained. Bone marrow aspirate concentrate (BMAC) contains other types of cells aside from stem cells. These cells contribute to the process of healing. Differences in content between BMAC and PRP are specified and the importance of adequate number and viability of stem cells is highlighted as one of crucial elements of their efficacy. The contents of the adipose tissue are discussed and the difference in number of stem cells between the bone marrow and adipose tissue is also mentioned. The studies comparing the efficacy of BMAC and adipose tissue are included.

Performing the collection of stem cells by using C arm and ultrasound are described in detail including potential risks. The necessary equipment and ingredients needed for collection are specified. Processing of extracted elements from the bone marrow or adipose tissue to get adequate concentration of stem cells is explained in detail.

The most frequent way of administration of stem cells is by injecting directly into the damaged structures. They can also be applied during arthroscopic or open surgeries. More complex way of application is by using biodegradable scaffolds. The ideal scaffold should be nonimmunogenic to the host, should support adhesions and ingrowth of cells as well as neovascularization and angiogenesis [1].

As a majority of sports injuries are treated conservatively, MSCs are usually injected directly to the injured tissues; tendons, ligaments, muscles, or joints. A most common source for young people with sports injuries is the bone marrow. The percentage of stem cells in the bone marrow is very small (0.001 to 0.01%) [2] and they are mixed with other cells like neutrophils, lymphocytes, eosinophil, monocytes, and basophils [3]. Bone marrow contains also growth factors and cytokines [2]. There is a large variation in quantity of platelets between individuals and accurate analysis of content is very important [4]. Considering the mixture of different cells, the term bone marrow aspirate concentrate (BMAC) is more precise and should be officially used. Comparative analysis of BMAC and PRP showed differences in the percentage of some cells and similarities in others. It was found that

S. Trebinjac, M. K. Nair, *Regenerative Injections in Sports Medicine*,
https://doi.org/10.1007/978-981-15-6783-4_12

BMAC contained more white blood cells, neutrophils, and platelets but a similar number of monocytes, lymphocytes, and eosinophils [5]. If performed properly, BMAC aspiration is a safe treatment [6]. The unresolved issue at the moment is the minimal number of viable stem cells to regenerate commonly injured mesenchymal structures. There are not enough studies to establish certain standards. Centeno and co-authors from Reggenexx, Colorado compared two groups of patients with knee osteoarthritis treated with different doses of bone marrow stem cells. The first group received the quantity of $\leq 4 \times 10^8$ and the second group received $>4 \times 10^8$. Both groups showed significant improvement but the group received a bigger quantity of cells experienced less post-treatment pain. There were no differences in other tested parameters [7].

Adipose tissue is another common source of stem cells and it might be more appropriate for elderly people because of larger quantities of cells compared to bone marrow. Previously, adipose tissue was considered as a store of energy and thermal insulator but latest researches show they have plenty of cytokines, transcriptional, and growth factors [8]. Also, it contains fibroblasts, monocytes, vascular smooth muscle cells, endothelial cells, macrophages, pre-adipocyte lymphocytes, and adipocyte stem cells (ADSC). It originates from mesoderm and can differentiate into adipocytes, chondrocytes, myocytes, osteoblasts, and neurocytes [9].Possibility of differentiation to chondrocyte and osteoblast makes adipose tissue alternative option to BMAC for treatment of sports injuries.

The important clinical issue is whether either of these two sources of stem cells has an advantage over the other one. The study conducted on patients with knee osteoarthritis showed positive outcomes from the baseline in both BMAC and adipose tissue groups without significant differences between them [10]. It is not clear whether the same effect is present in the sports population.

Some clinicians inject bone marrow and adipose tissue together assuming that it will provide better therapeutic effect. However, clinical study did not confirm additional benefits of such combination [11].

12.1 Collection of Stem Cells

The process of harvesting needs certain skills and practice. It is strongly recommended that it is performed under C arm or ultrasound guidance. This will reduce the risk of wrong placement of trocar.

To avoid any risk, a strict protocol must be followed. A procedure has to be conducted in aseptic conditions. The following are the most common equipments used for collection of Bone marrow stem cells:

1. Trolley for instruments
2. Syringes: 5 cc and 30 cc (alternative 10 cc)
3. Heparin
4. Phosphate buffered saline
5. Two sterile disposable trocars (one for each side)

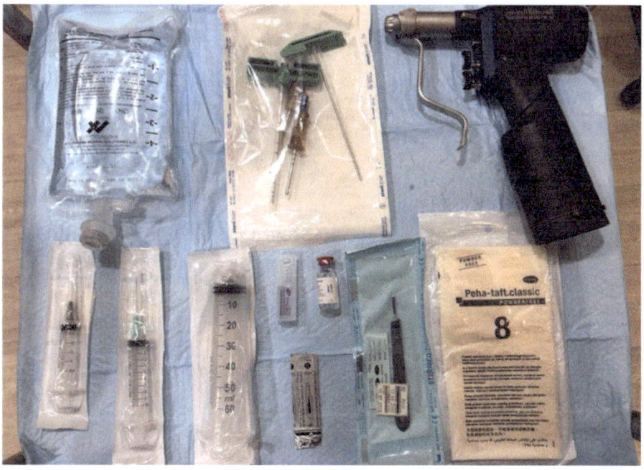

Fig. 12.1 Commonly used items for harvesting of BMAC

6. Small scalpel to cut the skin
7. Drill machine (optional) (Fig. 12.1)

12.2 BMAC Harvesting and Processing Technique

The procedure starts with positioning of patients in a prone or side position if the target of harvesting is the iliac crest. Alternative option is a supine position if the harvesting place is the anterior superior iliac spine. Whatever positions are used, it is important to make sure that the patient must feel comfortable.

The further description is related to the harvesting of BMAC from the iliac crest. Positioning of C arm fluoro is very important, it has to be focused on the posterior superior side of iliac crest from where the BMAC will be harvested. The image of the PSIS should be verified (Fig. 12.2).

Knowing anatomy in the area of trocar positioning is very important to avoid injury of the nerve and vascular structure. The attention should be paid to the location of cluneal nerves, gluteal artery, vein, and sciatic nerve. Penetration through the sacrum can cause serious complications (Fig.12.3).

The procedure must be performed in sterile conditions. The steps in performing procedure and processing BMAC are listed in Table 12.1.

The patient preparation is the same as for lower back surgical procedure (Fig. 12.4). Preferably the patient should be in conscious sedation. After disinfection with chlorhexidine, the skin is numbed with local anesthetic, usually Lidocaine 1%. The anesthetic should be applied to the subcutaneous tissue and periosteum. Under fluoroscopy, a trocar is inserted through the bone. After removing the stylet, 10 cc or 30 cc syringe is connected to the trocar. To prevent coagulation of the blood, 30,000 units of heparin is prepared in a syringe of 30 cc. For a 10 cc syringe it is 10,000 units of heparin. Bone marrow is extracted in small quantities of a few ml from different locations by changing the angle of the trocar or pushing the trocar deeper. Initial steps include palpation of iliac bone, local anesthesia and application of trocar (Fig. 12.5).

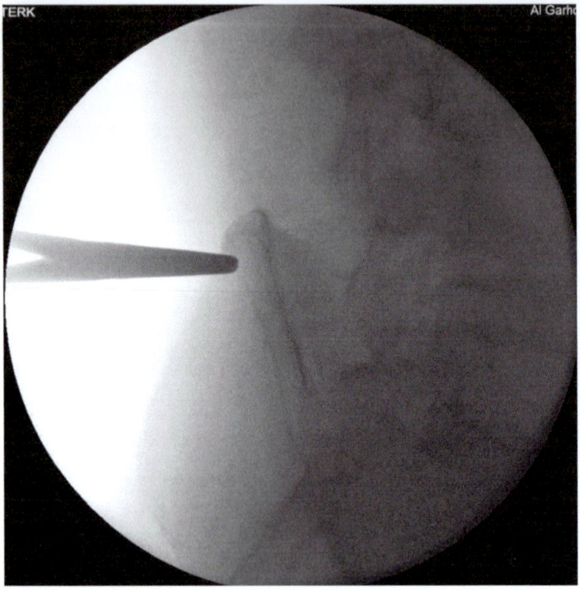

Fig. 12.2 PSIS, position where trocar is placed for harvesting of BMAC

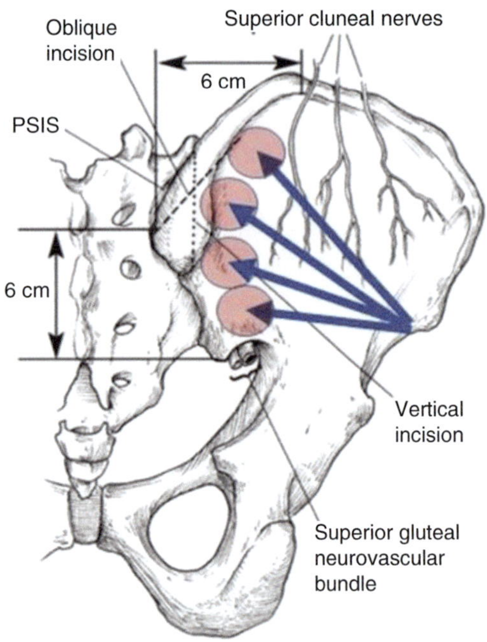

Fig. 12.3 Basic pelvic anatomy from [12] with permission

Table 12.1 Step-by-step process for harvest and processing of bone marrow aspiration

Step	Details
Patient positioning	Prone for PSIS harvest, supine for ASIS harvest
	Selection of anesthetic plan for aspiration
	Palpate site for aspiration
	Sterile preparation with antiseptic solution and sterile sheets/towels
Bone marrow aspiration	Confirmation of bony landmarks
	Injection of local anesthetic
	Preload aspiration syringe with 1 mL heparin (1000 U/mL)
	Insert aspiration trocar and needle through skin, down to bone
	Penetrate cortex with power tool
	Collection of 60 mL of bone marrow aspirate
Preparation of aspirate	Centrifuge according to the protocol, obtain approximately 6 mL BMAC sample
Application of aspirate	Select indication for injection (e.g., rotator cuff repair, revision ACL, osteoarthritis)
	Sterile preparation of selected injection site
	Injection of local anesthetic if selected for application
	Injection of aspirate in selected site

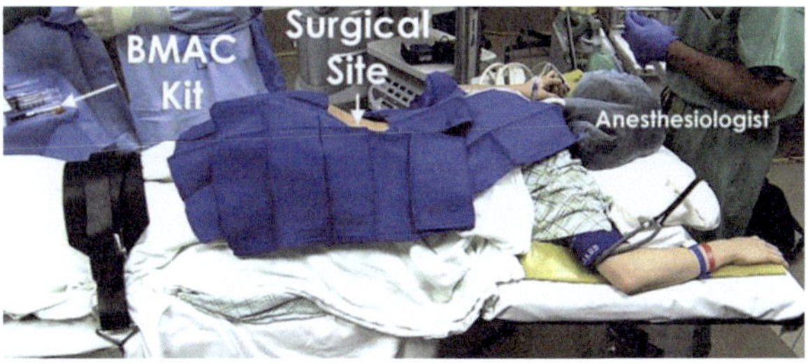

Fig. 12.4 The common set up for harvesting of BMAC: from [13] with permission

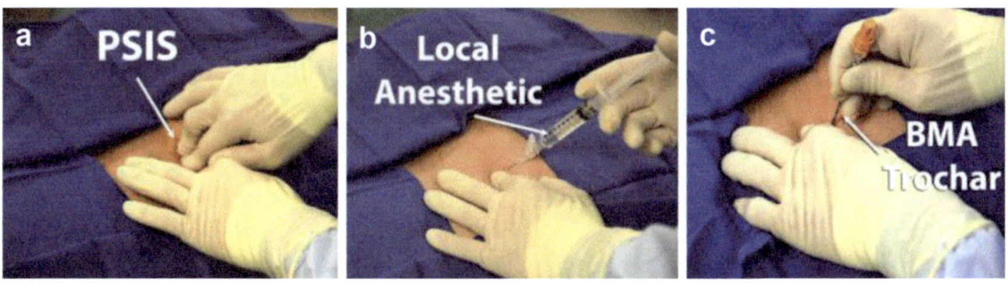

Fig. 12.5 (**a**–**c**) Steps in harvesting and processing of bone marrow aspirate from [13] with permission

Some physicians prefer to use a drill machine instead of a trocar to reduce mechanical pressure. For some patients, it might be less painful but the use of this machine needs certain skills by a practitioner and it is not recommended to be the first option for beginners (Fig. 12.6). The aspiration of bone marrow is presented in Fig. 12.7.

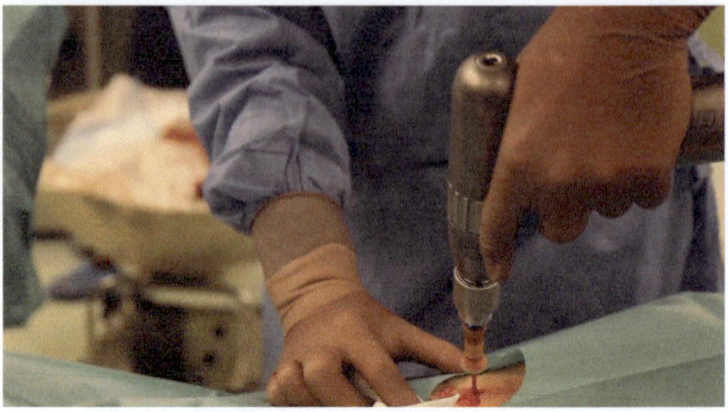

Fig. 12.6 Using a drill machine for BMAC collection

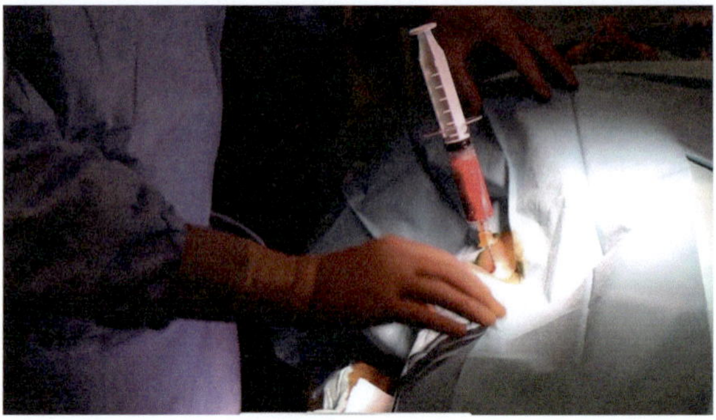

Fig. 12.7 BMAC aspiration

After BMAC is harvested it will be filtered and processed in the centrifuge machine to get concentrated products with MSCs and other ingredients. Unwanted elements like red blood cells will be removed (Fig. 12.8).

The number of cells should be counted by an automated cell counter. Aside from the number, it is important to know the percentage of viable cells. Quantity and quality of cells influence the therapeutic outcome [7].

If an ultrasound machine is used, instead of a C arm, then a low-frequency curvilinear probe has to be applied to the posterior side of the iliac bone. After identification of PSIS trocar is applied and bone marrow is harvested the same way as under the C arm.

12.3 Harvesting and Processing of Adipose Tissue

Harvesting stem cells from adipose tissue is considered an easier and less risky technique than bone marrow aspiration [14]. Depends on the part of the body from where fat is extracted, the patient can be in supine, prone, or side position. It is the personal decision of the doctor to decide the location of harvesting because there is no significant difference among the graft donated from the flank, upper and lower abdomen, inner or outer thigh [15]. Different methods of fat extractions are also tested including surgical resection, power-assisted liposuction (PAL), laser-assisted

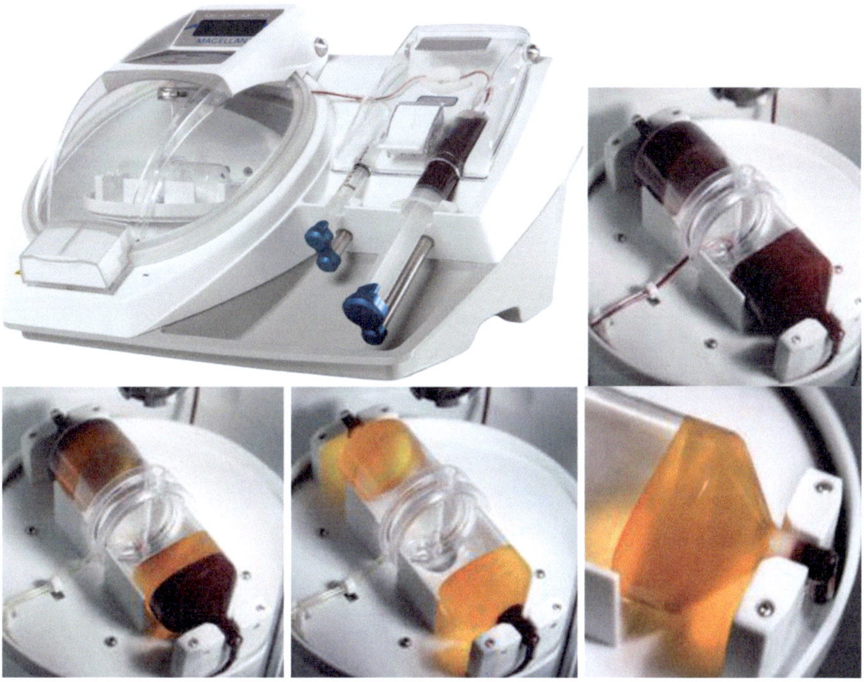

Fig. 12.8 Processing of BMAC in a centrifuge machine. Elimination of red blood cells. Image Courtesy Magellan Stem Cells

liposuction (LAL), or ultrasound-assisted liposuction (UAL). It was found that PAL technique is the best for clinical practice because of high proliferation and slow senescence of ASCs [16].

The procedure is a painful and tumescent solution consisting of sodium chloride, lidocaine or ropivacaine and epinephrine has to be prepared and delivered through cannula to the subcutaneous tissue. After providing good anesthesia and vasoconstriction of blood vessels (effects of epinephrine) the fat tissue is sucked to the syringe of 50 ml.

Lipoaspirate has to be proceeded by washing, digesting with enzyme and centrifuging to get a stromal vascular fraction (SVF) which contains ADSC, endothelial cells, endothelial precursor cells, T cells, macrophages, pericytes, preadipocytes, and smooth muscle cells [17]. Before application, some clinicians do in vitro analysis of SVF to get better insight into its contents and features.

In some countries the use of digestive enzymes is not allowed, considering it as more than minimal manipulation of stem cells, which might eventually modify their effect, eliciting adverse reactions. Also, enzyme digestion is an expensive and time-consuming process [18]. To avoid such obstacles mechanical forces are used for breaking adipose tissue and releasing ASCs [19] (Fig. 12.9). Diagram of harvesting, processing and analyzing of adipose stem cells is presented in Fig. 12.10.

While there is unbeatable evidence that bone marrow extract and adipose tissue generate vital stem cells, it is not the case with some other products. One of them is

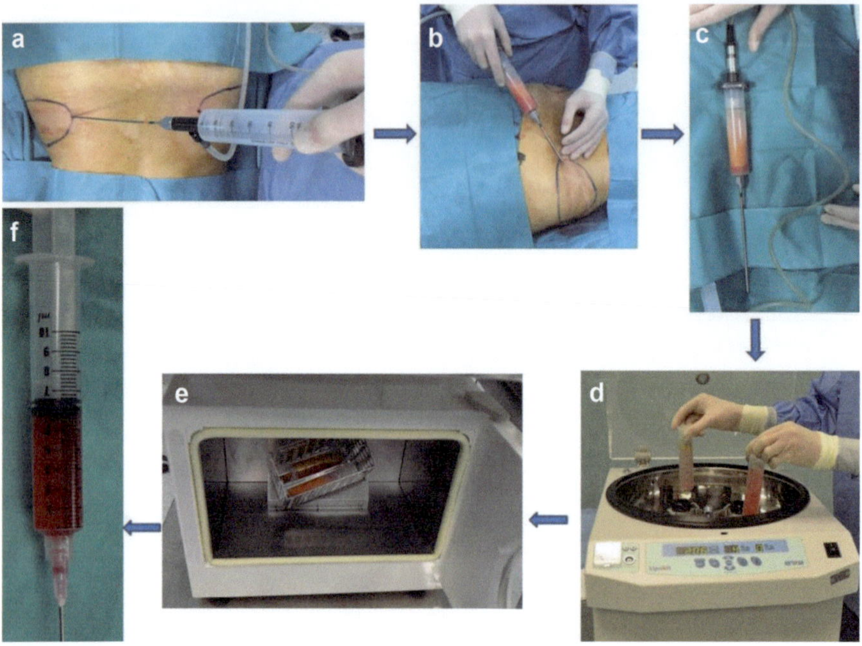

Fig. 12.9 (**a–f**) Steps in harvesting and processing of adipose tissue by using enzymes or mechanical force. Image Courtesy [20]

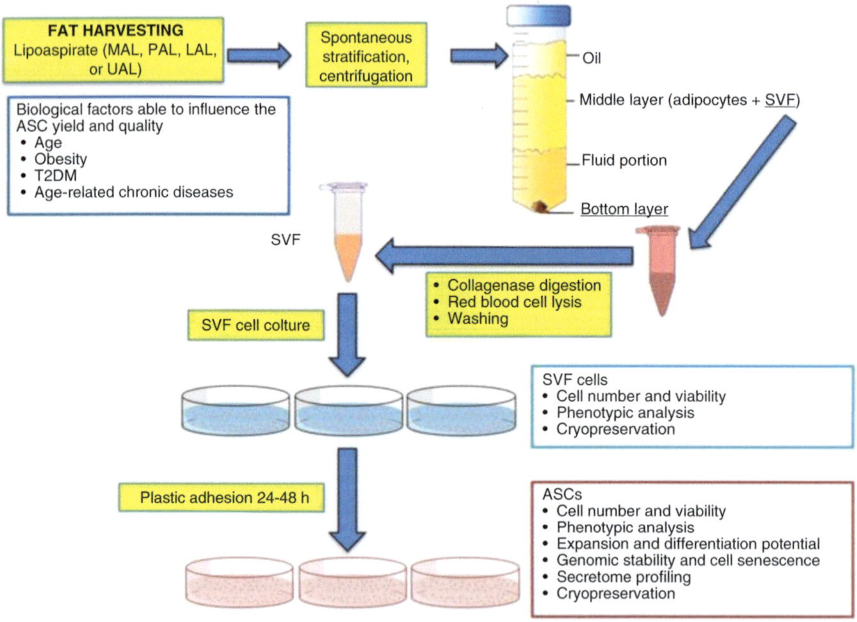

Fig. 12.10 Schematic presentation of harvesting, processing and analyzing adipose-derived stem cells from [13] with permission Creative Commons License

extracted from the amniotic and chorion part of placenta. It is an allogenic ready-made product mainly used for wound healing and in cosmetic purposes. Recently some studies showed promising results in the orthopedic field as well [21, 22]. Even though there is no evidence of functional stem cells, there are other ingredients that might stimulate regenerative processes. That is why these products are also included in the spectrum of regenerative therapy substances [21, 23]. However, the broad use of these products in sports medicine is still in an infantile stage.

Key Points

- Two most common sources of mesenchymal stem cells are bone marrow and adipose tissue.
- Bone marrow possesses a very small percentage of stem cells, much less than adipose tissue. Both tissues contain other ingredients with possible therapeutic effects.
- Comparative analysis between BMAC and PRP showed differences in percentage of some ingredients and similarities in others.
- The harvesting of BMAC should be performed under C arm fluoroscopy or ultrasound guidance. The use of heparin and local anesthetic is mandatory.
- Processing of bone marrow content is in a centrifuge machine to get concentrated samples for injection.
- Adipose tissue harvesting needs a tumescent solution for anesthesia and vasoconstriction.
- Processing of extracted fat could be either by using enzymes or by mechanical force.

References

1. Garzón I, Pérez-Köhler B, Garrido-Gómez J, Carriel V, Nieto-Aguilar R, Martín-Piedra MA, et al. Evaluation of the cell viability of human Wharton's jelly stem cells for use in cell therapy. Tissue Eng Part C Methods. 2012 Jun 1;18(6):48–419.
2. Holton J, Imam M, Ward J, Snow M. The basic science of bone marrow aspirate concentrate in chondral injuries. Orthop Rev. 2016 Sep 19;8(3):6659.
3. Bain B. The bone marrow aspirate of healthy subjects. Br J Haematol. 1996 Jul;94(1):206–9.
4. Mantripragada VP, Piuzzi NS, George J, Bova W, Ng M, Boehm C, et al. Reliable assessment of bone marrow and bone marrow concentrates using automated hematology analyzer. Regen Med. 2019 Jul 1;14(7):639–46.
5. Cassano J, Cassano J, Kennedy J, Kennedy J, Ross K, Ross K, et al. Bone marrow concentrate and platelet-rich plasma differ in cell distribution and interleukin 1 receptor antagonist protein concentration. Knee Surg Sports Traumatol Arthrosc. 2018 Jan;26(1):333–42.
6. Hendrich C, Franz E, Waertel G, Krebs R, Jäger M. Safety of autologous bone marrow aspiration concentrate transplantation: initial experiences in 101 patients. Orthop Rev. 2009 Oct 10;1(2):e32.
7. Centeno CJ, Al-Sayegh H, Bashir J, Goodyear S, Freeman MD. A dose response analysis of a specific bone marrow concentrate treatment protocol for knee osteoarthritis. BMC Musculoskelet Disord. 2015 Sep 18;16(1):258.
8. Kim EY, Kim WK, Oh K, Han BS, Lee SC, Bae K. Recent advances in proteomic studies of adipose tissues and adipocytes. Int J Mol Sci. 2015 Feb 27;16(3):4581–99.
9. Miana VV, González EAP. Adipose tissue stem cells in regenerative medicine. Ecancermedicalscience. 2018;12:822.

10. Mautner K, Bowers R, Easley K, Fausel Z, Robinson R. Functional outcomes following microfragmented adipose tissue versus bone marrow aspirate concentrate injections for symptomatic knee osteoarthritis. Stem Cells Transl Med. 2019 Nov;8(11):1149–56.
11. Centeno C, Pitts J, Al-Sayegh H, Freeman M. Efficacy of autologous bone marrow concentrate for knee osteoarthritis with and without adipose graft. Biomed Res Int. 2014;2014:370621–9.
12. Friedlis MF, Centeno CJ. Performing a better bone marrow aspiration. Phys Med Rehabil Clin N Am. 2016;27(4):919–39.
13. Chahla J, Mannava S, Cinque ME, Geeslin AG, Codina D, LaPrade RF. Bone marrow aspirate concentrate harvesting and processing technique. Arthrosc Tech. 2016;6(2):e441–5.
14. Palumbo P, Lombardi F, Siragusa G, Cifone MG, Cinque B, Giuliani M. Methods of isolation, characterization and expansion of human adipose-derived stem cells (ASCs): an overview. Int J Mol Sci. 2018 Jun 28;19(7):1897.
15. Li K, Li K, Gao J, Gao J, Zhang Z, Zhang Z, et al. Selection of donor site for fat grafting and cell isolation. Aesth Plast Surg. 2013 Feb;37(1):153–8.
16. Bajek A, Gurtowska N, Olkowska J, Maj M, Kaźmierski Ł, Bodnar M, et al. Does the harvesting technique affect the properties of adipose-derived stem cells?-the comparative biological characterization. J Cell Biochem. 2017 May;118(5):1097–107.
17. Bora P, Majumdar AS. Adipose tissue-derived stromal vascular fraction in regenerative medicine: a brief review on biology and translation. Stem Cell Res Ther. 2017 Jun 15;8(1):145–10.
18. Bellei B, Migliano E, Tedesco M, Caputo S, Picardo M. Maximizing non-enzymatic methods for harvesting adipose-derived stem from lipoaspirate: technical considerations and clinical implications for regenerative surgery. Sci Rep. 2017 Aug 30;7(1):10015.
19. Bianchi F, Maioli M, Leonardi E, Olivi E, Pasquinelli G, Valente S, et al. A new nonenzymatic method and device to obtain a fat tissue derivative highly enriched in Pericyte-like elements by mild mechanical forces from human Lipoaspirates. Cell Transplant. 2013 Nov;22(11):2063–77.
20. Raposio E, Simonacci F, Perrotta RE. Adipose-derived stem cells: comparison between two methods of isolation for clinical applications. Ann Med Surg. 2017 Aug;20:87–91.
21. Werber B. Amniotic tissues for the treatment of chronic plantar Fasciosis and Achilles Tendinosis. J Sports Med. 2015;2015:219896.
22. Gellhorn AC, Han A. The use of dehydrated human amnion/Chorion membrane allograft injection for the treatment of Tendinopathy or arthritis: a case series involving 40 patients. PM&R. 2017 Dec;9(12):1236–43.
23. Barboni B, Russo V, Curini V, Mauro A, Martelli A, Muttini A, et al. Achilles tendon regeneration can be improved by amniotic epithelial cell Allotransplantation. Cell Transplant. 2012;21(11):2377–95.

Clinical Applications of Stem Cells in Sports

13

The chapter starts with treatment in ligament and tendon lesions. A short narration of tendon healing stages and various tissue factors involved in the healing process are mentioned. Brief overview of how the ratio of type 1 to type 3 collagen changes as the healing progresses and the role played by the MSC in programming macrophages from type 1 to type 2 also given. Evidence for cellular changes for ligament and tendon healing in laboratory animal experiments are followed by human studies for clinical benefits. Effect of MSCs in osteoarthritis of Knee is also mentioned, even though the occurrence of it in early athletic life is rare. Limited number of high-quality studies in the sports field make it difficult to find systematic reviews and meta-analysis in MSC treatment.

The available literature for stem cell studies in the sports medicine field is sparse. The majority of studies were done in animals and most of the human clinical trials are for osteoarthritis of the knee.

13.1 Mesenchymal Stem Cell Treatment in Ligament and Tendon

13.1.1 Basic Principle

The normal process of healing for tendon and ligament rupture is to result in scar formation, which produces an inferior quality in structure and function compared with the original one. The process of healing in tendon and ligaments also involve the classical three stages of healing: Inflammation, proliferation, and remodeling. During the inflammatory stage, there is an infiltration of neutrophils, macrophages (M1 and M2), and lesser degrees of T lymphocytes occur in the wounded tissue. During proliferation, fibroblasts, endothelial cells, and macrophages accumulate resulting in granulation tissue. The number of type 3 collagen deposited is more compared to the type 1 collagen but weaker in strength than the type 1 [1].

S. Trebinjac, M. K. Nair, *Regenerative Injections in Sports Medicine*,
https://doi.org/10.1007/978-981-15-6783-4_13

Tenocytes are the basic cellular units of the tendon. They are made up of multiple molecules, of which type 1 collagen is the most dominant. Other minor collagen components are proteoglycans and glycoproteins. Type 3 collagen, tenascin, cartilage oligomeric matrix protein, and fibronectin are some of them. During tendon healing, tenocytes are found to deposit abundant type 3 collagen compared to type 1 [2]. In addition to type 1 collagen, there are other proteins and proteoglycans found to be essential in normal tendon differentiation. They are biglycan, decorin, fibromodulin, lumican, and tenomodulin [2]. Among these, biglycan and fibromodulin are thought to be critical in maintaining a niche for tendon progenitor cells [2].

When the healing progresses to the remodeling, the ratio of type 1 collagen increases. It is observed that healing closer to the original is attained through the early suppression of inflammatory cells and cytokines. The Mesenchymal Stem Cells program macrophages from M1 (pro-inflammatory) to M2 (anti-inflammatory) phenotype. The M2 macrophages found to reduce the area of tissue damage, reduce inflammation, act against M1 macrophages, and promote tissue repair [3]. The macrophages programmed by the MSCs are known as MSC educated Macrophages (MEM). The MEM expressed high levels of IL-10 and IL-6 and low levels of IL-12 and TNFα.

In vivo animal experiments, on rat medial collateral ligament, Chamberlain et al. [4] demonstrated that the phenotypic response is dose-dependent. Lower doses of MSCs ($1x10^6$) produced a low inflammation due to fewer M1 macrophages compared with higher doses (4×10^6). According to their findings, tendons treated with preconditioned MSCs (to be more anti-inflammatory) shown to be having more strength than the nonconditioned one. Macrophages polarize into 2 phenotypes depending upon the cytokine exposure in their environment. When they are exposed to inflammatory cytokines like IFNγ and TNFα they polarize to M1 phenotype, which are inflammatory in nature and produce more inflammatory cytokines and free radicals. These are thought responsible for scarring and fibrosis. Whereas when they are exposed to anti inflmmatory cytokines like IL-4 and 13 they polarize to M2 macrophages which are anti-inflammatory in nature, which produce anti-inflammatory cytokines like IL-10, IL-1 Ra, TGFβ. These are thought to be responsible for regeneration. Pro inflammtory and anti-inflammatory substances are presented in Fig. 13.1.

Chamberlain et al. found that Mesenchymal Stromal Stem Cells are capable to polarize macrophages into M2 type by paracrine mechanisms. They also observed co-culturing of CD14+ macrophages with MSCs resulted in M2 like macrophages. Very recently they could generate M2 like macrophages from extracellular vesicles isolated from MSCs, also known as Exosome Educated Macrophages (EEM). In their experiments on mouse Achilles tendon rupture model, treatment with EEM showed improved mechanical properties, reduced inflammation, and earlier angiogenesis.

According to the study conducted by Ouyang et al., allogeneic bone marrow stromal cells implanted to rabbit patellar tendon could survive for about 8 weeks and able to differentiate into tenocyte-like cells 5 weeks after implantation [5].

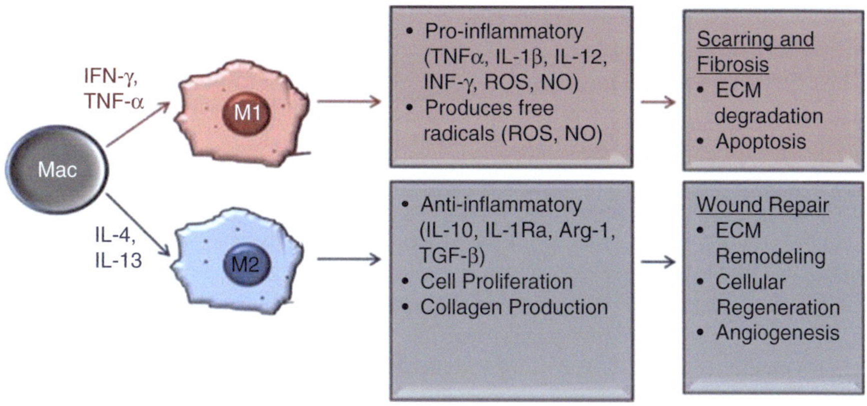

Fig. 13.1 MSC producing pro- or anti-inflammatory properties: Source [4] Creative Commons

In another study on rabbit patellar tendons treated with autologous bone marrow mesenchymal stem cells, showed significant improvement in maximum stress, strain, energy density due to an increase in the number of cells and quantity of mature collagen fibers. But injecting undifferentiated bone marrow MSCs found to produce ectopic bone formation in the tendons [6].

Experiments done in rat medial collateral ligament injury found local upregulation of stromal cell-derived factor – 1 and correlated systematically induced bone marrow stromal cells. According to the experiments done by Shimode et al., SDF-1 was temporarily upregulated with a peak reaching 2 weeks after the injury and homing rate of the systematically induced bone marrow stromal cells temporarily peaked 2–4 weeks after injury, proving that SDF-1 played a crucial role in homing of the stem cells [7]. Observations made by Tellier et al. after injecting with localized SDF-1 α on rat supraspinatus tendon injury model, found about fourfold increase in anti-inflammatory M2 macrophages and threefold increase in MSCs compared with the one treated without SDF-1α [8].

The role of adipose-derived mesenchymal stem cells in tendon repair is limited [9].

Skin-derived tenocyte-like cells were studied for the treatment of patellar tendinopathy, compared with autologous plasma. The study was a randomized control trial including 60 tendons. The patients were assessed for pain severity and function with the VISA score (Victorian Institute of Sports Assessment). Ultrasound assessments were done to evaluate tendon thickness, neovascularity, hypoechogenicity, intrasubstance tears. The study showed improved VISA score and faster improvement in the cellular group [10].

Tendon Derived Stem Cells (TDSC) are relatively recent isolation and shown to have clonogenicity, self-renewal, and multilineage differentiation capacity similar to MSCs [11]. Bi et al. identified tendon resident stem cells, termed Tendon Derived Stem Progenitor Cells (TSPCs) [12]. The function of TSPCs found to decline with aging, disease, and injury. Wang et al. studied the efficacy of ultrasound-guided autologous tenocyte injection (ATI) in patients with refractory lateral epicondylitis. These patients were followed up for 4.5 years for improvement in clinical function and evaluated with MRI tendinopathy scores. The majority of the patients (93%) were satisfied with the treatment and MRI evidence showed improvement in the mean grade of tendinopathy. Even though it was a case series study, long term follow-up with imaging and scoring were the strengths of this study [13].

Trials with intratendinous injection of the adipose-derived stromal vascular fraction (SVF) into Achilles tendon was found to be safe and efficacious treatment by Usuelli et al. The study was a randomized controlled trial with 6 months follow-up. SVF injection was compared with the PRP group. Both the groups showed an improvement, but the SVF arm showed significant improvement in 15 and 30 days time indicating it a faster result. The difference eased out in later stages of the trial [14].

In a systematic review of stem cell treatment of tendons in humans, Haiko et al. found no evidence [15]. But this review was having a lot of limitations as it included all types of studies- randomized and non-randomized trials, cohort, and case series. Only one study was randomized and three were case series. They included 4 published and 3 unpublished/pending trials. They did not have data for unpublished trials. The studies were non-homogenous as it included both bone marrow and adipose-derived stem cells. One study included culturing and the other 3 were not having a culture. The number of cells was variable. All the studies show some form of improvement, but since the risk of bias is high, the authors concluded there is no evidence for the treatment.

13.2 Mesenchymal Stem Cells in Patellar Tendinopathy

In a 5 year follow up of five patients with chronic patellar tendinopathy, Pascual-Garrido et al. found that bone marrow mononuclear cells (BM-MNC) could produce statistically significant changes [16].

13.3 Mesenchymal Stem Cells in Osteoarthritis

There was limited evidence for adipose-derived stem cells (ADSC) (in the form of Stromal Vascular Fraction (SVF) in Knee osteoarthritis, according to a systematic review by Hurley et al. [17]. Of the 14 studies evaluated for knee, the majority used PRP, fibrin, or PRP + fibrin in addition to SVF. Five studies mentioned 90% satisfaction and none reported any complications related to liposuction. There is a probability of confounding due to the use of other biologicals along with ADSC.

In a systematic review with the GRADE approach, Hirotaka et al. observed that mesenchymal stem cell treatment significantly improved knee pain and self-reported function in patients with knee OA. They also found MSC treatment significantly improves cartilage quality in some studies but the quality of evidence was very low to low according to the GRADE approach [18].

Munar A et al. conducted a case series study on the treatment of knee OA by expanded autologous bone marrow mesenchymal stem cells. The study included 50 clinical cases and results are verified by MRI before and after treatment [19].

A hundred ml of bone marrow was aspirated from the iliac crest of patients and sent to the lab for selection and culture. The expansion time was about 22 days and obtained 113×10^9 mononuclear cells and 40×10^6 MSC. These cells were suspended in 8 ml of suspension and applied as an intra-articular infusion. Clinical evaluation was done with VAS, Lequesene, and WOMAC indices prior to treatment and at 6 and 12 months after treatment. The cell viability was measured with a Neubauer camera and found to be 85%. Cartilage assessment was done with T2 mapping average values (ms). Altogether 88 regions of interest (ROI) were defined in patellar cartilage, femoral condyle, and tibial plateau. The T2 relaxation times were averaged for each area and poor cartilage index (PCI) estimated as the percentage of T2 values >50 ms. PCI 100 is the worst possible value and value near 5 considered healthy. They found the mean PCI significantly decreased from 25 to 5 at 12 months after injection. The decrease in PCI found in 74% of patients [19].

Key Points

- The process of tendon healing involves classical three stages.
- Tenocytes are the basic cellular units of tendons and they are predominant in type 1 collagen.
- In the initial stages of healing, the number of type 3 collagen is higher than type 1, but as the healing progresses, type 1 becomes predominant.
- Mesenchymal stem cells program macrophages from pro-inflammatory type (M1) to anti-inflammatory (M2) phenotype.
- Rat experiments show that the phenotypic response is dose-dependent, a lower dosage of MSC produces low inflammation due to fewer M1 macrophages, and tendons pre-treated with MSC are shown to be having more strength.
- The evidence for adipose-derived stem cells' role in tendon repair is limited.
- Systematic reviews of stem cell treatments in tendons for humans did not show encouraging results.
- Evidence for ADSC in osteoarthritis of the knee is limited.
- MSC from autologous bone marrow in osteoarthritis of the knee shows promising results.

References

1. Oreffo R, Bennett A, Carr A, Triffitt J. Patients with primary osteoarthritis show no change with ageing in the number of Osteogenic precursors. Scand J Rheumatol. 1998;27:415–24.
2. Liu C, Aschbacher-Smith L, Barthelery N, Dyment N, Butler DL, Wylie C. What we should know before using tissue engineering techniques to repair injured tendons: a developmental biology perspective. Tissue Eng. 2011 Jun;17(ja):165.
3. Chamberlain CS, Clements AEB, Kink JA, Choi U, Baer GS, Halanski MA, et al. Extracellular vesicle-educated macrophages promote early Achilles tendon healing. Stem Cells. 2019 May;37(5):652–62.

4. Chamberlain CS, Saether EE, Aktas E, Vanderby R. Mesenchymal stem cell therapy on tendon/ligament healing. J Cytokine Biol. 2017 May;2(1):112.
5. Ouyang HW, Goh JCH, Lee EH. Viability of allogeneic bone marrow stromal cells following local delivery into patella tendon in rabbit model. Cell Transplant. 2004 Sep;13(6):649.
6. Awad HA, Butler DL, Boivin GP, Smith FN, Malaviya P, Huibregtse B, et al. Autologous Mesenchymal stem cell-mediated repair of tendon. Tissue Eng. 1999 Jun;5(3):267–77.
7. Shimode K, Iwasaki N, Majima T, Funakoshi T, Sawaguchi N, Onodera T, et al. Local Upregulation of stromal cell–derived Factor-1 after ligament injuries enhances homing rate of bone marrow stromal cells in rats. Tissue Eng A. 2009 Aug 1;15(8):2277–84.
8. Tellier L, Krieger J, Brimeyer A, Coogan A, Falis A, Rinker T, et al. Localized SDF-1α delivery increases pro-healing bone marrow-derived cells in the supraspinatus muscle following severe rotator cuff injury. Regen Eng Transl Med. 2018 Jun;4(2):92–103.
9. Obaid H, Connell D. Cell therapy in tendon disorders. Am J Sports Med. 2010 Oct;38(10):2123–32.
10. Clarke AW, Alyas F, Morris T, Robertson CJ, Bell J, Connell DA. Skin-derived Tenocyte-like cells for the treatment of patellar Tendinopathy. Am J Sports Med. 2011 Mar;39(3):614–23.
11. Lui P, Chan K. Tendon-derived stem cells (TDSCs): from basic science to potential roles in tendon pathology and tissue engineering applications. Stem Cell Rev Rep. 2011 Nov;7(4):883–97.
12. Li L, Inkson CA, Seo B, Zhang L, Young MF, Shi S, et al. Identification of tendon stem/progenitor cells and the role of the extracellular matrix in their niche. Nat Med. 2007 Oct;13(10):1219–27.
13. Wang A, Mackie K, Breidahl W, Wang T, Zheng MH. Evidence for the durability of autologous Tenocyte injection for treatment of chronic resistant lateral Epicondylitis. Am J Sports Med. 2015 Jul;43(7):1775–83.
14. Usuelli F, Grassi M, Maccario C, Vigano M, Lanfranchi L, Alfieri Montrasio U, et al. Intratendinous adipose-derived stromal vascular fraction (SVF) injection provides a safe, efficacious treatment for Achilles tendinopathy: results of a randomized controlled clinical trial at a 6-month follow-up. Knee Surg Sports Traumatol Arthrosc. 2018 Jul;26(7):2000–10.
15. Pas HIMFL, Moen MH, Haisma HJ, Winters M. No evidence for the use of stem cell therapy for tendon disorders: a systematic review. Br J Sports Med. 2017;51(13):996–1002.
16. Cecilia P-G, Rolón A, A. Makino. Treatment of chronic patellar Tendinopathy with autologous bone marrow stem cells: a 5-year-Followup. Stem Cells Int. 2012;2012:953510–5.
17. Hurley E, Yasui Y, Gianakos A, Seow D, Shimozono Y, Kerkhoffs G, et al. Limited evidence for adipose-derived stem cell therapy on the treatment of osteoarthritis. Knee Surg Sports Traumatol Arthrosc. 2018 Nov;26(11):3499–507.
18. Iijima H, Isho T, Kuroki H, Takahashi M, Aoyama T. Effectiveness of mesenchymal stem cells for treating patients with knee osteoarthritis: a meta-analysis toward the establishment of effective regenerative rehabilitation. NPJ Regen Med. 2018;3(1):15–3.
19. Munar A, Soler Rich R. Treatment of knee osteoarthritis with autologous expanded bone marrow Mesenchymal stem cells: 50 cases clinical and MRI results at one year follow-up. J Stem Cell Res Therapy. 2015;5(6):285–91.

14 Rehabilitation After Regenerative Injection procedures

This section gives an overview of Rehabilitation after regenerative injections, mainly for PRPs as the principles remain the same for PRP and MSC. Posttreatment rehabilitation is essential in athletes for an early return to sports. This prevents the recurrence of injury and prepares the athletes for full functional recovery. Rehabilitation after regenerative injections is given paramount importance that a separate terminology was coined "Regenerative Rehabilitation". An account of Regenerative Rehabilitation is given along with an explanation of the importance of mechanotransduction in the differentiation of stem cells. Stage wise rehabilitation after regenerative injections in osteoarthritis of the knee is explained. Two different rehabilitation protocols after PRP injections for patellar tendinopathy are compared. We could not find any specific protocols in literature for post-injection rehabilitation after bone marrow/ adipose-derived stem cell injections.

In order to get the full benefit of regenerative medicine treatments, it is essential to have a structured rehabilitation program after the regenerative procedures.

The patients sustaining an injury and suffering from pain are most of the time candidates for regenerative injection therapy. Since pain is an inhibitor of muscle function, it is always associated with loss of function and muscle power. Most of these patients would be having impaired proprioception along with muscle weakness. So all regenerative injection treatments in musculoskeletal conditions should be followed up with rehabilitation programs.

Rehabilitation is closely associated with regenerative medicine to the extent of developing a new terminology "Regenerative Rehabilitation."

It is defined as *"the synergistic integration of principles and approaches from the regenerative medicine and rehabilitation fields, with the goal of optimizing form and function as well as patient independence"* [1].

Regenerative medicine or rehabilitation approaches provide a foundation for the restoration of tissue architecture, promotion of organ function, reduction of disability, or improvement of quality of life. However, it is the combination of both approaches working synergistically that can optimize or maximize the individual functional outcome [1].

S. Trebinjac, M. K. Nair, *Regenerative Injections in Sports Medicine*,
https://doi.org/10.1007/978-981-15-6783-4_14

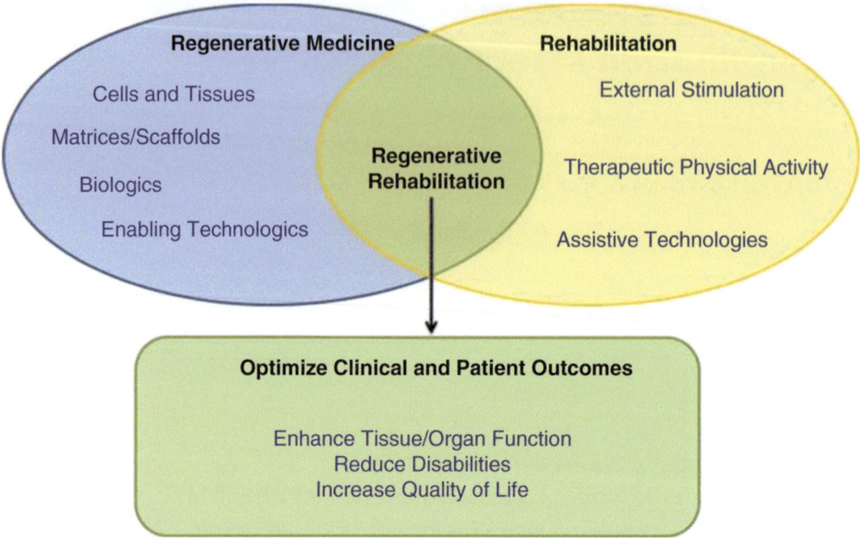

Fig. 14.1 Regenerative Rehabilitation: adapted from [1] with permission

Regenerative rehabilitative strategies may include activity-mediated plasticity, exercise dosing, electrical stimulation, proprioceptive rehabilitation, sports specific exercises, and endurance building measures. Each and every case would be having critical barriers, which has to be taken into consideration while incorporating regenerative medicine techniques into clinical practice. The main areas from rehabilitation realm to be considered are functional capacities, goals of patient and physician (achievable or not), range of motion, sensation, and pain (Fig. 14.1).

Application of mechanotransduction principles in regenerative medicine is a useful tool in achieving better outcomes. There is a constant communication between stem cells and their local microenvironment (niche) through mechanical cues to regulate cell fate, cell behavior, and guiding developmental processes. Mechanical stimuli are found to be involved in organogenesis and patterning in embryonic development. Mechanical cues are important in pluripotent stem cells for differentiation and mechanical and physical cues are important in adult cells in maintaining potency [2].

Mechanotransduction can be endogenous or exogenous. Intrinsic forces are generated intracellularly also called cell-generated forces. These forces are transferred to other cells through cell to cell junction receptors or traction on extracellular matrix ligands. The transduction of the mechanical cues depends upon the elastic modulus of the extracellular matrix. Extrinsic forces are the forces that are applied externally by shear, tension, or compression on cells. The cytoskeleton transfers these forces from membrane protein to the nucleus, where it influences gene expression and cellular behavior [2].

The human chondrocytes are found to be affected by mechanical stimuli. The mechanical features of the joint articular microenvironment, such as hydrostatic pressure, shear, and compressive forces promote stem cell differentiation to chondrocytes [3]. In addition to mechanical stimuli, local bioelectrical signals also found

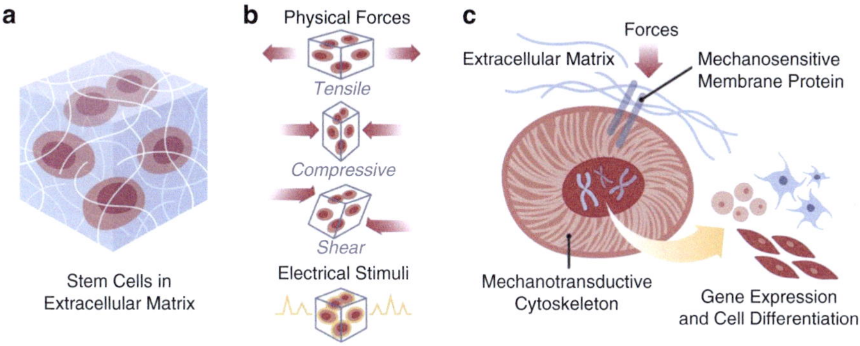

Fig. 14.2 Schematic diagram explaining how mechanotransduction promotes cell differentiation: adapted from [3] with permission

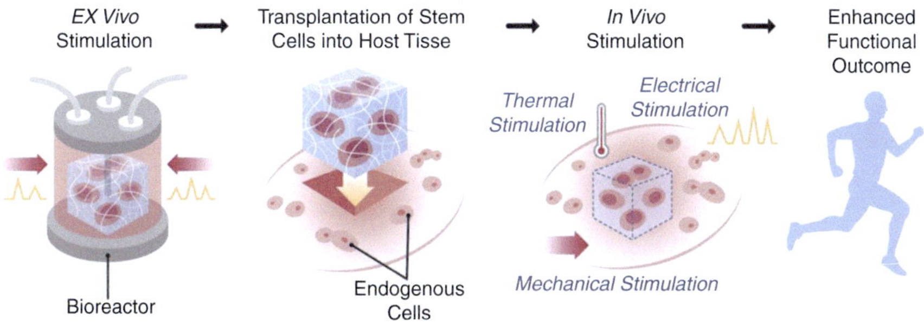

Fig. 14.3 Schematic diagram shows how rehabilitation therapies stimulates mechanotransduction which in turn enhance functional outcomes: adapted from [3] with permission (**a**) Stem Cells are embedded in its own local mileu and extracellular matrix which exert biophysical pressure. (**b**) Biophysical pressures are Physical stimuli (viz tensile and compressive forces and shear) and electrical stimuli from neural cells and local fields. (**c**) The cells responds to these stimuli by trasnducing these signal from the cell membrane to the nucleus through cytoskeleton, which influences the gene expression and cell differentiation

to influence cells. Electrical stimulations found to be effective in promoting axonal outgrowth, nerve regeneration and skin wound healing by directing cellular migration by endogenous electrical currents [3] (Fig. 14.2).

Rehabilitation principles include tissue and joint loading by means exercise prescriptions, application of tensile forces through stretching, joint mobilization, and traction, electrical stimulation by electrotherapy and compression and rarefaction and heating by ultrasound. These therapies are found to be effective in enhancing functional outcomes after injury in integumentary, neuromuscular, neurological, and musculoskeletal systems [3] Using biophysical principles, Stem cells can be manipulated *exvivo* to enhance its transplantation efficacy. Using rehabilitation therapies, both transplanted cells and the host environment can be manipulated *invivo* fostering stem cell growth and differentiation. Rehabilitation approaches like exercises and stretching produces mechanical stimulation, transcutaneous electrical stimulation produces electrical stimulation and application of heat or cold produces thermal stimulation (Fig. 14.3).

Like rehabilitation medicine, regenerative medicine is also not restricted to any organ systems. The main aim of rehabilitation is the restoration of function according to the potential of the patient considering his impairment. Similarly, regenerative medicine tries early restoration of function through cellular regeneration at a microscopic level.

Rehabilitation medicine and regenerative medicine are complementary and mixing these two sciences would help sportspeople to enhance functional recovery.

As the use of regenerative medicine in various sports conditions is quite recent, there are not many scientifically validated protocols available in literature. Most of the research is done in Osteoarthritis of the knee. But the incidence of osteoarthritis is rare in Sportspeople in their earlier careers. Most of them develop it as a consequence of injury and at a later stage of their life. Since the volume of literature available for Osteoarthritis and Regenerative Medicine is so vast, it is inappropriate not to mention it in this context.

Rehabilitation protocols in knee osteoarthritis after regenerative injections (Table 14.1).

14.1 Rehabilitation After Platelet Rich Plasma Injection for Patellar Tendinopathy

A simplified version of rehabilitation protocol for Platelet Rich Plasma injections in patellar tendinopathy can be obtained from Mauntner et al. [5].

According to this protocol, the rehabilitation is divided into 3 phases (Table 14.2).

According to a review of literature by Kaux JF et al., the rehabilitation protocol is longer for chronic jumper's knee after PRP injection, which lasts up to 52 weeks post-injection [6]. The details of the program are as follows.

In the first week after PRP injection, the patient has to have relative rest, cryotherapy, and pain killers if needed to relieve pain, but not NSAIDs as it might interfere with platelet function. Patients can participate in his activities of daily living as usual.

In the second week after injection, can start isometric exercises 3 sessions of 15 repetitions, eccentric exercises with knee bend at 45 degree angle, 3 sessions of 15 repetitions three times a week, electromyostimulation, quadriceps stretching, and cryotherapy.

In the third week of the program, the number of isometric strengthening and eccentric exercises is increased from 3 sessions of 15 repetitions to 5 sessions of 15 repetitions and the addition of low resistance cycle ergometer for 10 min. The rest of the program is the same as in week two; electromyostimulation, quadriceps stretching, and cryotherapy.

In week four, the cycle ergometer exercise duration and resistance remain the same. The isometric strengthening of the quadriceps is set at 5 sessions of 20 repetitions and eccentric exercises are done with knee bend at 60°, instead of 45° and 3 sessions of 20 repetitions, three times a week. The rest of the therapy programs remain the same as in the third week.

Table 14.1 Rehabilitation protocol knee osteoarthritis after regenerative injections; adapted with permission from [4]

	Day 0–3 immediate post-intervention	Day 3–14 posttreatment	2–4 weeks posttreatment	5–10 weeks posttreatment
Goals	Protect area treated and pain control when required Range of motion (ROM) to tolerance Promote healing Patient education about KOA and weight management Improve joint mobility	Increase local circulation Increase tissue tolerance through exercise or rehab Improve muscular strength and endurance Progress to full ROM. Avoid deconditioning Ongoing patient education weight management as needed Precautions: Deep squatting, twisting, kneeling, closed chain deep knee flexion activities	Progress muscular strength and endurance training Open chain versus closed chain Initiate balance and proprioception training on stable surfaces Patient education about KOA and weight management Initiate aquatic therapy	Improve muscular strength and endurance Progress balance and proprioception to unstable surfaces Patient education about KOA and weight management Precautions: Avoid impact activities Continue modalities PRN

(continued)

Table 14.1 (continued)

	Day 0–3 immediate post-intervention	Day 3–14 posttreatment	2–4 weeks posttreatment	5–10 weeks posttreatment
Precautions	No activity that causes pain	Weight-bearing and exercises as tolerable		
Suggested therapeutic modality/exercises	Passive joint and soft tissue mobilization techniques Gentle active ROM exercises Address swelling (manual lymphatic drainage) Isometrics above and below treated area If joint ROM is restricted due to pain, taping and/or bracing may be warranted Electro modalities: LLLT (total dose equal to or greater than 27 J); TENS//IFC as required for pain management Acupuncture to surrounding periarticular structures	Passive joint and soft tissue mobilization techniques Graded load progression with active ROM exercises Gradually increase intensity of isometrics above and below treated area (core/hip/knee strengthening) Electro modalities: LLLT (total dose equal to or greater than 27 J); TENS/IFC as required for pain management Acupuncture to surrounding periarticular structures WBV therapy (frequency of 35–40 Hz, vibration 60 s, interval rest 60 s) in combination with squat Water exercise- whole body movements, with warm up, stretching/flexibility component and cool down. Weight-assisted treadmill	Graded load progression with active ROM exercises + stretching exercises Continued strengthening exercises (core/hip/knee strengthening) + implement eccentric exercises Dynamic exercises with Thera band resistance band Proprioceptive, neuromuscular and stability training LLLT (total dose equal to or greater than 27 J) TENS/IFC as required for pain management Initiate static loading exercises- wall squat holds, leg press holds, mini squat holds, etc. WBV therapy (frequency of 35–40 Hz, vibration 60 s, interval rest 60 s) in combination with squat BFRT- perform 4 sets (30, 15, 15, 15 repetitions) at 15–30% of 1RM. Cuff placement as proximal as possible on involved limb Water exercise- increase intensity and/or duration of water-based exercises.	• Graded load progression with active ROM exercises + stretching exercises. • Advance closed chain exercises- leg press, squats, step up/down, etc. • Continued progressive strengthening exercises (core/hip/knee strengthening). • High-intensity resistance exercise. • Good eccentric and concentric loads that are multi-planar. • LLLT (total dose equal to or greater than 27 J). TENS/IFC as required for pain management WBV therapy (frequency of 35–40 Hz, vibration 60 s, interval rest 60 s) in combination with squat BFRT- perform 4 sets (30, 15, 15, 15 repetitions) at 15–30% of 1RM. Cuff placement as proximal as possible on involved limb Water exercise- increase intensity and/or duration of water-based exercises. Progress static loading to greater degrees of knee flexion

Cardiovascular exercises	None	Cycling, swimming, walking- low impact aerobic exercise. Can be accumulated in bouts of 10 min, aim for 150 min/week		
Progression criteria	Pain and swelling are controlled ROM is maintained	Pain and swelling are controlled ROM is maintained Gait is normalized	Pain and swelling are controlled ROM is maintained Pain-free muscle testing	Pain and swelling are controlled ROM is maintained Good dynamic neuromuscular control with multi-plane activities and without pain

If increased pain, return to the previous step until pain is controlled and full return to function required for that step.
Abbreviations: *KOA* knee osteoarthritis, *ROM* range of motion, *PRN* pro re nata, (as circumstances require) *LLLT* low-level laser therapy, *TENS* transcutaneous electric nerve stimulation, *IFC* interferential current, *WBV* whole-body vibration, BFRT blood flow restriction therapy

Table 14.2 Rehabilitation protocol for PRP injections—patellar tendinopathy: adapted from with permission [5]

Phase	Length of Time	Restrictions	Rehabilitation
Phase1: Tissue protection	Days 0–3	Consider NWB or protected WB for lower extremity procedures, especially if in pain. No weight training, avoid NSAIDs and use limited ice	Relative rest. Activities as tolerated; avoiding excess loading or stress to the treated area. Gentle AROM
Phase 2: Early tissue healing, facilitation of collagen deposition	Days 4–14	Progress to FWB without a protective device. Avoid NSAIDs	Light activities to provide motion to the tendon; aerobic exercise that avoids loading of the treated tendon. Gentle prolonged stretching. Begin treatment on kinetic chain/adjacent regions. Glutei strengthening and core strengthening
	Weeks 2–6	Avoid eccentric exercises. Avoid NSAIDs. Avoid ice	Progress to WB activities. Low weight, high repetition isometrics (pain scale <3/10). OKC activities. Soft tissue work to tendon with CFM, IASTM, and "dynamic" stretching
Phase 3: Collagen strengthening	Weeks 6–12		Eccentric exercises (keep pain scale <3/10). Two sets of 15 repetitions. CKC activities. Plyometrics; proprioceptive training and other sport-specific exercises. Progress to WB activities and consider a return to sport if pain <3/10
	Months 3+	Reassess improvement; if not >75% improved consider repeat injection and return to phase I	Progress back to functional sport-specific activities with increasing load on tendon as pain allows

AROM Active range of motion, *CFM* Cross-friction massage, *CKC* Closed kinetic chain, *FWB* Full weight-bearing, *IASTM* Instrument-assisted soft tissue mobilization, *NWB* Non-weight bearing, *OKC* Open kinetic chain, *WB* Weight-bearing

In the fifth week of the program, the intensity of cycle ergometry increased to moderate resistance level to 10 min. In addition to the other components, proprioception is added as a new thing this week. Eccentric exercises increased to 5 sessions instead of 3.

In the sixth week, the main change is increasing knee flexion to 90 degrees for eccentric exercises and sessions reduced to 3.

In the seventh week of post-injection, cycle ergometry is done with high resistance for 10 min, eccentric exercises are done in an inclined plane of 25 degrees with the knee at 60 degrees bending, 3 sessions of 20 repetitions, three times a week. The isometric exercises are done at the same repetitions as in previous weeks.

From 8 weeks to 12 weeks the intensity of eccentric exercises increased from 3 to 5 sessions of 20 repetitions, three times a week without physical therapist supervision and re-athletisation (a function of the sport) with patellar taping or bracing. The strengthening of quadriceps, quadriceps stretching, and cryotherapy continues.

From 13th week onward till the end of the rehabilitation program (52 weeks), eccentric exercises on an inclined plane, knee flexion increased to 90° and with 20 repetitions for 5 sessions, two times a week without physical therapist supervision. Sports after warming-up and with patellar taping or bracing. Stretching of the quadriceps and cryotherapy to be continued [6] (Table 14.3).

Table 14.3 Rehabilitation protocol after PRP injections for Chronic Patellar tendinopathy: Adapted from [6]

Weeks since injection	Rehabilitation		
			New additions/ changes from previous week
First week	Cryotherapy	Relative rest with activities of daily living allowed Painkillers if needed *No NSAIDs*	
Second week	Cryotherapy, electromyostimulation Quadriceps stretching	Quadriceps isometric strengthening exercises: *15 reps × 3 sessions* Eccentric exercises (knee bend *45 degrees*): *15 repetitions × 3 sessions*—3 times/ week	Quadriceps Isometric strengthening exercises: *15 reps × 3 sessions* Eccentric exercises (knee bend *45 degrees*): *15 repetitions × 3 sessions*—three times/ week Electromyostimulation and Quadriceps stretching
Third week	Cryotherapy, electromyostimulation Quadriceps stretching	Quadriceps Isometric strengthening exercises: *15 reps × 5 sessions* Eccentric exercises (knee bend *45 degrees*): *15 repetitions* × *5* sessions—three times/ week Cycle Ergometry; low resistance 10 min	Cycle Ergometry; *low resistance 10 min* *Exercises sessions increased to 5 from 3*
Fourth week	Cryotherapy, electromyostimulation Quadriceps stretching	Quadriceps Isometric strengthening exercises: *20 reps × 5 sessions* Eccentric exercises (knee bend *60 degrees*): *20 repetitions* × 3 sessions—three times/ week Cycle ergometry; *low resistance 10 min*	*Exercises increased to 20 repetitions* *Knee flexion increased to 60 degrees*

(continued)

Table 14.3 (continued)

Weeks since injection	Rehabilitation		
			New additions/ changes from previous week
Fifth week	Cryotherapy, electromyostimulation Quadriceps stretching	Quadriceps Isometric strengthening exercises: *20 reps × 5 sessions* Eccentric exercises (knee bend *60 degrees*): *20 repetitions* × *5* sessions—3 times/ week Cycle Ergometry; *moderate resistance 10 min* *Proprioceptive exercises*	*Proprioceptive exercises* Cycle ergometry; *moderate resistance*
Sixth week	Cryotherapy, electromyostimulation Quadriceps stretching	Quadriceps Isometric strengthening exercises: *20 reps × 5 sessions* Eccentric exercises (knee bend *90 degrees*): *20 repetitions* × 3 sessions—three times/ week Cycle Ergometry; *moderate resistance 10 min* *Proprioceptive exercises*	*Knee flexion increased to 90 degrees*
Seventh week	Cryotherapy, electromyostimulation Quadriceps stretching	Quadriceps Isometric strengthening exercises: *20 reps × 5 sessions* Eccentric exercises *25 degree inclined plane* (knee bend *60 degrees*): *20 repetitions × 3* sessions—three times/ week Cycle Ergometry; *high resistance 10 min* *Proprioceptive exercises*	Eccentric exercises *in inclined plane* with less knee bend with less number of sessions (three sessions) Cycle Ergometry; *high resistance*
Eighth to twelveth week	Cryotherapy, Quadriceps stretching	Quadriceps Strengthening exercises Eccentric exercises *25 degree declined board* (knee bend *60 degrees*): *20 repetitions* × *3–5* sessions—three times/ week *without PT supervision* *Re-athletisation (function of the sport) with patellar taping or bracing*	*Eccentric exercises in declined board* *Eccentric exercises without PT supervision* *Re-athletisation (function of the sport) with patellar taping or bracing* *Electromyostimulation, Cycle ergometry, proprioceptive exercises discontinued*

Table 14.3 (continued)

Weeks since injection	Rehabilitation		
			New additions/ changes from previous week
Thirteen to fifty-two week	Cryotherapy, Quadriceps stretching	Eccentric exercises *inclined plane* (knee bend *90 degrees*): *20 repetitions* × *5* sessions—*two times/* week *without PT supervision as warming up Sports with patellar taping or bracing*	Eccentric exercises in inclined plane without PT supervision knee bend 90 degrees two times/ week *Sports after warming-up and with patellar taping or bracing*

According to the protocol by M van Ark et al. [7] rehabilitation of patellar tendinopathy after PRP injections is divided into 5 phases.

The Phase 1 is inflammation and proliferation which might last up to 2 weeks. Phase 2 is proliferation, which is from second to fourth week. The third phase 3 is the remodeling phase in weeks 5 and 6. From the seventh to eighth week is the Integration Phase. Phase 5 is sports specific after eighth week. The details of these phases can be found in the table below. Table 14.4.

14.2 Return to Play Decisions

Returning to sports decisions after treatment is not simple, and vary depending upon many factors. It will be different for the same medical condition but for different athletes in different sports. Even for athletes participating in the same sports with the same intensity, the decision to return to play will be different. A three-step decision-based Return To Play (RTP) model was developed by Creighton, Shrier, Shultz, Meeuwisse, Matheson [8]. According to them, RTP decision depends upon three factors; health status, participation risk, and decision modification. The first process is to do risk evaluation and it includes evaluation of health status and participation risk. Evaluation of health status is the first step and medical factors of athletes such as patient demographics, symptoms, medical history, signs, lab tests, functional tests, psychological status, and other potentially serious medical factors like concussion are taken into consideration.

Table 14.4 Rehabilitation Phases after PRP injections for patellar tendinopathy. From [7] with permission

Phase 1—inflammation/proliferation phase (0–2 weeks)
Inform and advise patient, rest, low load (1x week physical therapy)
Day 1–3 inform and advise patient
• Rest
• Low load (walk with two crutches)
• Reduce pain (cryotherapy)
Day 4–7 inform and advise patient
• Optimize ROM if necessary, combined with isometric exercises for quadriceps muscle
• Increase ADL with VAS pain score < 50
Day 7–14 exercise
• optimize knee flexion and extension combined with unloaded cycling (home trainer).
• Walking: 100% load without crutches.
• Home exercise program: quadriceps muscle isometric contraction, active straight-leg raise, abduction side-lying (2× day, 3 × 20 reps., rest interval 30–60 sec).
Pain score must not exceed 50 on the VAS scale during all exercises and activities of daily living.
Phase 2—proliferation phase (weeks 2–4)
More dynamic and active exercises (1×2 weeks physical therapy)
• Higher cycling intensity (build up load), goal: 20–30 min.
• Home exercise program:
– Squats, calf extensions, single-leg squat with arm swing, abduction side-lying. Cycling on home trainer. (3 × 20 reps, rest interval 30-60 sec.)
– Exercises have to be possible (need to be executed) in complete ROM.
– Closed chain exercises, mainly coordination and strength endurance. Stability plays no major role yet.
– Light pain (VAS < 50) allowed during exercises, however the pain must decrease after the exercise.
Phase 3—remodeling phase (weeks 5, 6)
Active exercises are expanded (2× week physical therapy).
• Eccentric exercises are integrated into the program.
Home exercise program (on days without supervised physical therapy): 2 days/week single-leg squat on decline board (25°).
• Various exercises (strength endurance) to increase load capacity of lower extremity, including home trainer warm-up, core stability exercises, lunges, abduction side-lying, squats, and step-downs (3×15 reps., rest interval 30 sec).
• Integrate core stability exercises (e.g., prone bridge, side bridge).
A pain increase within 48 h is allowed (VAS < 50), but the pain must have disappeared after 48 h. No leg extension in open chain.
Phase 4—integration phase (weeks 7, 8)
Exercises progressing to higher %1RM, 3 × 8–15 reps., rest interval 30 sec, more muscular hypertrophy (2× week physical therapy)
• Daily eccentric training (2× day, 3 × 20 reps.).
• Run-and-walk exercises of increasing intensity and difficulty (starting with interval walking/jogging, advancing to multidirectional, acceleration, and deceleration running).
• Jump exercises with increasing difficulty. (correct execution with controlled landing important. Start with height jumps, progress to long jumps.)
• Core stability with higher difficulty.

(continued)

Table 14.4 (continued)

• Sport-specific exercises at maximal and speed strength.
Phase 5—Sport-specific phase (after eighth week)
• Daily eccentric training continues (2× day, 3×20 reps.) until end of supervised physical therapy program (±12 weeks).
• Advance to more sport-specific exercises, e.g., plyometric, a-lactic, multidirectional running, acceleration, and deceleration.

ADL Activities of Daily Living, *reps.* repetitions, *ROM* Range Of Motion, *sec.* seconds; *VAS* Visual Analog Scale

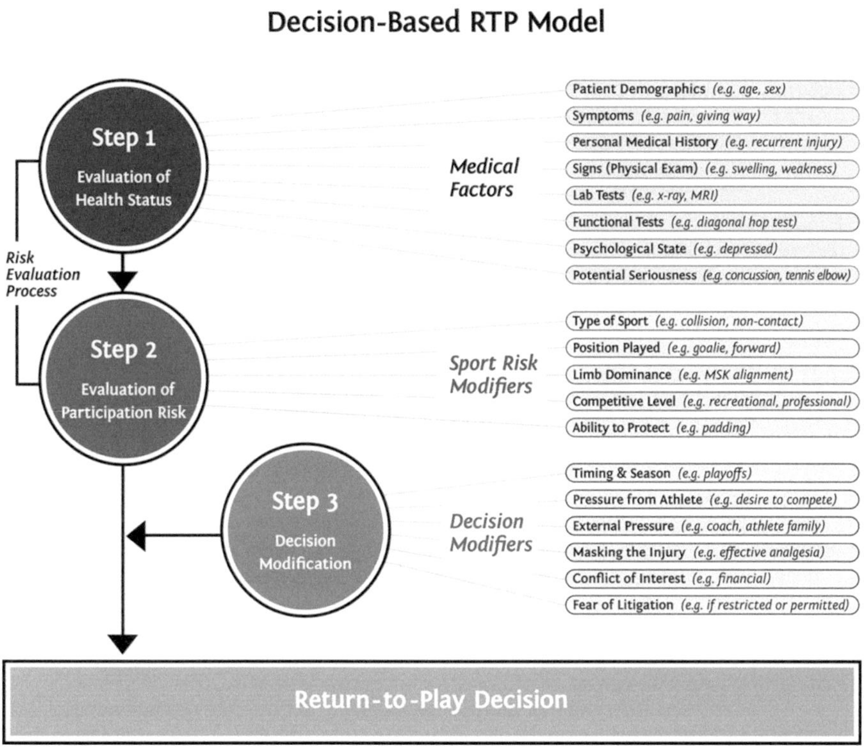

Fig. 14.4 Adapted from [8] with permission

In the second step, participation risk is evaluated and risk factors pertaining to sports like the type of sport, the position of a player, limb dominance, competition level, and ability to protect is taken into account.

The third and final step is to have decision modification by considering various factors like timing and season, pressure from the athlete and coach or club to compete, fear of litigation and conflict of interest (Fig. 14.4).

Key Points

- Regenerative rehabilitation is a new field.
- Regenerative medicine and rehabilitation are mutually complementary.
- Mechanotransduction found to be important in the differentiation of stem cells.
- Regenerative Rehabilitation found to enhance functional recovery in athletes.
- The protocol for rehabilitation after regenerative injections in osteoarthritis of the knee could extend up to 10 weeks post-injection.
- Protocols for rehabilitation after PRP injections in patellar tendinopathy differ in duration: According to Mauntner et al., there are 3 phases and lasts for 3 months. The protocol by Kaux et al. lasts for 52 weeks. Protocols by M van Ark et al. spreads in 5 phases and last more than 12 weeks.
- We could not find any specific rehabilitation protocols post-injection bone marrow/adipose-derived stem cells.
- Return to play decision is not simple and a three step model was proposed for supporting the return to play decision.

References

1. Rose LF, Wolf EJ, Brindle T, Cernich A, Dean WK, Dearth CL, et al. The convergence of regenerative medicine and rehabilitation: federal perspectives. NPJ Regenerative medicine. 2018;3(1):19–7.
2. Vining KH, Mooney DJ. Mechanical forces direct stem cell behaviour in development and regeneration. Nature reviews. Mol Cell Biol. 2017 Dec;18(12):728–42.
3. Rando TA, Ambrosio F. Regenerative rehabilitation: applied biophysics meets stem cell therapeutics. Cell Stem Cell. 2018 Mar 1;22(3):306–9.
4. McKay J, Frantzen K, Vercruyssen N, Hafsi K, Opitz T, Davis A, et al. Rehabilitation following regenerative medicine treatment for knee osteoarthritis-current concept review. J Clin Orthop Trauma. 2018;10(1):59–66.
5. Mautner K, Malanga G, Colberg R. Optimization of ingredients, procedures and rehabilitation for platelet-rich plasma injections for chronic tendinopathy. Pain Manag. 2011 Nov;1(6):523–32.
6. Kaux J, Forthomme B, Namurois M, Bauvir P, Defawe N, Delvaux F, et al. Description of a standardized rehabilitation program based on sub-maximal eccentric following a platelet-rich plasma infiltration for jumper's knee. Muscles Ligaments Tendons J. 2014 Jan;4(1):85–9.
7. van Ark M, van den Akker-Scheek I, Meijer LTB, Zwerver J. An exercise-based physical therapy program for patients with patellar tendinopathy after platelet-rich plasma injection. Phys Ther Sport. 2013;14(2):124–30.
8. Creighton D, Shrier I, Shultz R, Meeuwisse W, Matheson G. Return-to-play in sport: a decision-based model. Clin J Sport Med. 2010 Sep;20(5):379–85.

The Future of Regenerative Medicine 15

The prevalence of musculoskeletal injuries is significantly high and it will increase in the future. It might cause an additional economic burden to society. This chapter discusses the possible directions of development of dextrose prolotherapy, PRP, and mesenchymal stem cells. It is assumed that regenerative medicine will become an important part of clinical practice in managing musculoskeletal conditions. It will be particularly involved in the rehabilitation of sports injuries. The importance of a better understanding of the possible actions of regenerative substances is highlighted. The need for comparative studies among three treatment modalities as well as increasing the number of randomized control trials is mandatory to enrich evidence-based practice. It was pointed out that ethical consideration and strict regulations play a very important role in the future implementation of regenerative substances.

It is accounted that one of two persons in the USA suffers at least one of around 150 diagnoses related to the musculoskeletal system. The prevalence is comparable to combined cardiovascular and respiratory disorders together. The costs of treatment in 2011 in the USA exceeded 213 billion US$ [1]. The number of people participating in different sports increasing and the same is with the number of musculoskeletal injuries. Considering the mentioned facts we can expect a big economic burden caused by chronic musculoskeletal conditions in the near future.

Regenerative medicine has the potential to dramatically change the treatment outcome of many diseases and injuries. Inner body capacity to restore the morphology and function will eliminate the need for organ transplantation. The rehabilitation period after sports injury will be reduced and athletes will be able to extend their professional careers. The number of surgical interventions will be reduced.

However, this ideal scenario is not around the corner. Scientists involved in laboratory and animal research together with clinicians face complex challenges. The question addressed for a long time has been related to the mechanism of action of stem cells, platelet-rich plasma, and dextrose ingredients. This is a crucial issue that needs to be solved for more efficient therapeutic outcomes.

S. Trebinjac, M. K. Nair, *Regenerative Injections in Sports Medicine*,
https://doi.org/10.1007/978-981-15-6783-4_15

Dextrose prolotherapy can be a good alternative option for the management of sports injuries. It was proved to be safe and cost-effective. Athletes are usually in good general condition with fewer co-morbidities. Their immunological system is strong and the therapeutic response more favorable than in the general population. By reducing pain and strengthening damaged ligaments, tendons and joints, prolotherapy can reduce the recovery period and return people back to training and competition.

Dextrose prolotherapy must focus on a better understanding of the effect of different concentrations of dextrose in the treatment of chronic tendinosis, ligament, muscle, and joint injuries and degenerative diseases. Proinflammatory versus anti-inflammatory mechanisms of action have to be elucidated. We need to understand the possible role of growth factors and other molecules involved in the healing cascade. What is the optimal concentration for different tissues and each individual? What is the optimal treatment protocol? How many injections are enough and how often do they need to be injected? Experimental studies in vitro and in vivo should demonstrate real regenerative potential and remodeling of injected tissues.

Randomized control trials to compare dextrose prolotherapy injections with more known procedures like PRP and stem cells are very important to clarify the place of dextrose injections in the broad spectrum of regenerative substances.

The advantage of dextrose therapy is its low price, easy and simple preparation, and very high safety profile. Unfortunately, interest in further research is much less than for other regenerative substances. At the moment there are only six research projects registered at the website clinicaltrials.gov related to dextrose prolotherapy, of which one is terminated. Out of the remaining five studies, four are clinical and only one will measure inflammatory modulators trying to explain a possible mechanism of actions of hypertonic dextrose. Until pharmaceutical corporations invest in the more scientific exploration of this natural ingredient, dextrose injections will remain as a subject of interest for clinicians and future development will be based on their own research and practical experience.

Platelet-rich plasma (PRP) is obviously a more attractive subject for research because under these terms there are 353 research projects registered at the clinicaltrials.gov. It is observed that the field of interest is expanding more and more. In orthopedic and sports medicine recent concern is shifting from injecting peripheral joints to spine management. Several articles presented the effect of PRP on lumbar disk disorder [2, 3, 4]. Also, different non-musculoskeletal conditions have been treated with PRP [5, 6].

The subjects of further investigations will be the role of growth factors and other substances in the process of angiogenesis, immunomodulation, and synthesis of extracellular matrices.

At the moment there is no consensus among the scientists related to the role of leukocyte added to platelets, single or double spinning, frequency of treatment, the total number of repetitions. Differences in therapeutic outcomes are probably related to the composition of substances and how they are applied [7].

Lack of serious side effects and adverse reactions, at least in short-term applications is one of the most important arguments for widespread use of PRP. However, there is missing information related to the long-term consequences. More clinical studies are needed to compare PRP with dextrose prolotherapy and stem cells as separate injections or in combination.

There is no doubt that the biggest interest in the field of regenerative medicine is related to stem cells. The website clinicaltrials.gov registered 5320 research papers focused on their investigation. Such a huge number is not only an indicator of enormous interest but also illustrates the shortage of firmly established scientific facts related to their real effect. As stem cells are extracted from different sources and have different features, it is necessary to understand the characteristics of each type of cell in a term of their efficacy but also potentially dangerous side effects. Embryonic cells and induced pluripotent cells offer unprecedented regenerative potential but at the same time bear the risks of dangerous reactions. Reprogramming processes to convert adult fibroblast cells into iPSCs face already certain obstacles because only 0.1–3% of transfected cells become iPSCs [8, 9]. The hurdles are also related to inefficiency, incomplete reprogramming, and possible mutations of the cells [10]. However, in spite of not resolving issues, research of iPSCs moved from pre-clinical studies to clinical application in humans. The first human application was for the treatment of macular degeneration, age-related vision impairment. The patient reported improvement in visual acuity without any adverse reactions [11]. The University in Kyoto announced the first clinical trial on the application of iPSCs for the treatment of Parkinson's disease [12]. The team from Mayo clinic announced recently significant motor and sensory recovery of tetraplegic patients after the application of adipose-derived stem cells [13]. While there are some other clinical trials on the way no one is related to sports medicine at the moment.

The mesenchymal stem cells will probably be the main focus of sports injuries management. Since being discovered around 30 years ago, their intensive research resulted in around 55,000 publications available so far [14]. Our understanding of engrafting, intercellular signaling, and paracrine functioning is constantly progressing but it is still insufficient to explain all complexity of stem cells. The proliferating process in vitro does not replicate in vivo in the same way because the fate of stem cells is very much dependent on the environment by which they are surrounded. One of the most important research objectives is to decode the interaction of stem cells with their environment. The role of extracellular elements, exosomes, and microvesicles are the subjects of investigation because bioactive molecules, like growth factors and cytokines, are contained in these structures [15, 16]. Their function will provide better insight into paracrine effects of stem cells. There is a trend of injecting certain anti-inflammatory biomolecules like cytokines and selected growth factors rather than full volume of PRP, BMAC, or fat tissue. Whether it will provide more benefits is not clear at the moment. Also, individually designed therapy is of great interest to scientists and pharmaceutical industries.

The ethical issues and legislative regulation will be of main concern in the field of regenerative medicine. At the moment it is still an unregulated market and there is a lack of consensus about the best practice. The shortage of high-quality trials and comparative studies between different substances attributed as a regenerative, reinforcing the "gray zone" and individual (mis)interpretations. Companies advertising their products looking for revenue before scientifically established facts. The work on protocols and guidelines is much needed and must correlate with clear clinical evidence. Laboratory research in vitro and in vivo should integrate the knowledge of molecular biology, cytology, and genetics to better understand extremely complex characteristics of molecules that might have regenerative potential.

Injection administration will be the mainstay approach to the management of sports injuries. Most of them are treated conservatively and the procedure can be easily applied in outpatient clinics. The regenerative injections probably will be an integrative part of rehabilitation programs and will gradually minimize the use of corticosteroids and pain killers. Returning to sport in the shortest possible time remains the most important goal in professional sport and regenerative therapy is the frontrunner in its realization. However, the solid evidence that injection of dextrose prolotherapy, PRP, or mesenchymal stem cells really reduces the time of recovery and returning back to play is missing at the moment. The evaluation of such a possibility should be one of the priorities in further research.

Key Points

- The number of sports injuries increasing followed by increased costs of their treatment.
- Regenerative medicine will be a part of common practice in sports rehabilitation.
- Advantage of dextrose prolotherapy is high safety and low price. Mechanism of action, optimal concentration, and unified protocol of treatment need to be investigated in the future.
- Exploring the role of growth factors will be one of the priorities in the research of PRP.
- Paracrine effect, signaling system and engrafting are processes that need further elaboration for better understanding of the functioning of mesenchymal stem cells.
- The ethical issues and legislative regulations will need strict implementation in research and clinical practice of regenerative medicine.

References

1. Briggs AM, Woolf AD, Dreinhöfer K, Homb N, Hoy DG, Kopansky-Giles D, et al. Reducing the global burden of musculoskeletal conditions. World Health Organization. Bull World Health Organ. 2018 May 1;96(5):366–8.
2. Tuakli-Wosornu YA, Terry A, Boachie-Adjei K, Harrison JR, Gribbin CK, EE LS, et al. Lumbar Intradiskal platelet-rich plasma (PRP) injections: a prospective, double-blind, randomized controlled study. PM&R. 2016 Jan;8(1):1–10.
3. Platelet-rich plasma (PRP) and disc lesions: a review of the literature. Neuro-Chirurgie. 2017 Dec 1;63(6):473–7.
4. Monfett M, Harrison J, Boachie-Adjei K, Lutz G. Intradiscal platelet-rich plasma (PRP) injections for discogenic low back pain: an update. Int Orthop (SICOT). 2016 Jun;40(6):1321–8.
5. Elghblawi E. Platelet-rich plasma, the ultimate secret for youthful skin elixir and hair growth triggering. J Cosmet Dermatol. 2018 Jun;17(3):423–30.

6. Dawood AS, Salem HA. Current clinical applications of platelet-rich plasma in various gynecological disorders: an appraisal of theory and practice. Clin Exp Reprod Med. 2018 Jun;45(2):67–74.
7. Milano G, Sánchez M, Jo CH, Saccomanno MF, Thampatty BP, Wang JH. Platelet-rich plasma in orthopaedic sports medicine: state of the art. J ISAKOS: Joint Disord Orthop Sports Med. 2019 Jul;4(4):188–95.
8. Apostolou E, Hochedlinger K. Chromatin dynamics during cellular reprogramming. Nature. 2013 Oct 24;502(7472):462–71.
9. Yamanaka S, Hong H, Kanagawa O, Nakagawa M, Okita K, Ichisaka T, et al. Suppression of induced pluripotent stem cell generation by the p53-p21 pathway. Nature. 2009 Aug 27;460(7259):1132–5.
10. Takahashi K, Yamanaka S. A decade of transcription factor-mediated reprogramming to pluripotency. Nature reviews. Mol Cell Biol. 2016 Mar;17(3):183–93.
11. Fritsche LG, Fariss RN, Stambolian D, Abecasis GR, Curcio CA, Swaroop A. Age-related macular degeneration: genetics and biology coming together. Annu Rev Genomics Hum Genet. 2014 Aug 31;15(1):151–71.
12. Stoddard-Bennett T, Reijo PR. Treatment of Parkinson's disease through personalized medicine and induced pluripotent stem cells. Cells. 2019 Jan;8(1):26.
13. Bydon M, Dietz AB, Goncalves S, Moinuddin FM, Alvi MA, Goyal A, et al. CELLTOP clinical trial: first report from a phase 1 trial of autologous adipose tissue–derived Mesenchymal stem cells in the treatment of paralysis due to traumatic spinal cord injury. Mayo Clin Proc. 2019 Nov;95(2):406–14.
14. Pittenger MF, Discher DE, Péault BM, Phinney DG. Mesenchymal stem cell perspective: cell biology to clinical progress. NPJ Regen Med. 2019 Dec 2;4:22.
15. Phinney DG, Pittenger MF. Concise review: MSC-derived Exosomes for cell-free therapy. Stem Cells. 2017 Apr;35(4):851–8.
16. Börger V, Bremer M, Görgens A, Giebel B. Mesenchymal stem/stromal cell-derived extracellular vesicles as a new approach in stem cell therapy. ISBT Sci Ser. 2016 Jan;11(S1):228–34.

Index

S. Trebinjac, M. K. Nair, *Regenerative Injections in Sports Medicine*,
https://doi.org/10.1007/978-981-15-6783-4

MIX
Papier aus verantwortungsvollen Quellen
Paper from responsible sources
FSC® C105338

If you have any concerns about our products,
you can contact us on
ProductSafety@springernature.com

In case Publisher is established outside the EU,
the EU authorized representative is:
Springer Nature Customer Service Center GmbH
Europaplatz 3, 69115 Heidelberg, Germany

Printed by Libri Plureos GmbH
in Hamburg, Germany